# EYECARE BUSINESS

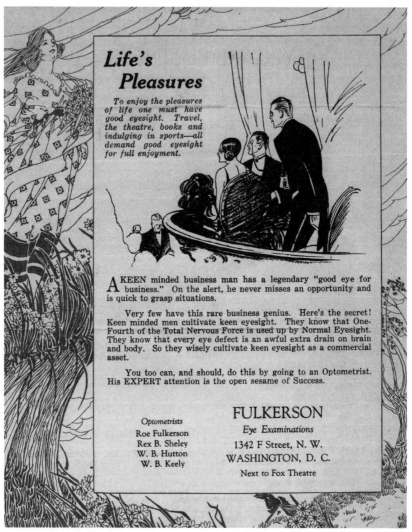

The earliest piece of direct mail known to the authors, used by an optometrist c.1920. It was a three-part-folded stamped mailing.

# EYECARE BUSINESS

## Marketing and Strategy

### Gary L. Moss, O.D., M.B.A., F.A.A.O.

Associate Professor of Community Care and Public Health,
New England College of Optometry, Boston;
Adjunct Instructor, Emmanuel College, Boston

### Peter G. Shaw-McMinn, O.D.

Assistant Professor of Clinical Science,
Southern California College of Optometry,
Fullerton

*Foreword by*
Barry J. Barresi, O.D., Ph.D.

Vice President for Clinical Care and Services and
Professor of Health Policy,
New England College of Optometry, Boston

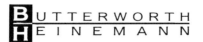

Boston   Oxford   Auckland   Johannesburg   Melbourne   New Delhi

**Library of Congress Cataloging-in-Publication Data**

Moss, Gary L.
  Eyecare business : marketing and strategy/Gary L. Moss, Peter G. Shaw-McMinn.
    p. cm.
  Includes bibliographical references and index.
  ISBN 0-7506-7238-2 (alk. paper)
  1. Ophthalmology—Marketing.   I. Shaw-McMinn, Peter.   II. Title.
RE72 .M67 2001
617.7'0068'8—dc21                                                              00-049806

**British Library Cataloguing-in-Publication Data**

A catalogue record for this book is available from the British Library.

The publisher offers special discounts on bulk orders of this book.
For information, please contact:

> Manager of Special Sales
> Butterworth-Heinemann
> 225 Wildwood Avenue
> Woburn, MA 01801-2041
> Tel: 781-904-2500
> Fax: 781-904-2620

For information on all Butterworth–Heinemann publications available, contact our World Wide Web home page at: http://www.bh.com

10 9 8 7 6 5 4 3 2 1

Printed in the United States of America

# Contents

# Foreword

The publication of *Eyecare Business: Marketing and Strategy* is a milestone in the education of the eyecare business clinician. The student resident and practicing doctor seeking success in today's dynamic health care marketplace now has a textbook that meets the competitive challenges of the future. For the first time in eyecare, one book blends the seasoned experience of successful practitioners with contemporary knowledge of management science.

Drs. Gary Moss and Peter Shaw-McMinn have the right stuff: quality care clinicians with business savvy able to teach their colleagues the management pearls of success. I have the benefit of firsthand knowledge of their talents since I served on the faculty of both Peter's academic home at the Southern California College of Optometry and Gary's teaching base at the New England College of Optometry. I remember Peter's successful early efforts in practice management teaching and curriculum development in the 1980s. In the mid-1990s, Gary was a bundle of intellectual energy as he was in the midst of his MBA studies, actively publishing management articles, and already plotting out his vision for a series of practice management textbooks.

Gary and Peter are truly experts to be respected and should be revered for translating the essence of their experience and knowledge into this text on strategic management. Expertly addressing the topics of market research and strategic planning for all levels of clinical experience, this text gives the student resident, new practitioner, and later-career doctors a sound foundation for practice building and business development in eyecare.

This is a book to study, explore, reread and, most impor-
tantly, help you learn each day on the frontline of patient care and
health care business. It is the first substantive text, seeped in the
science of today's MBA programs, which serves the sophisticated
information needs of today's eyecare business clincian. This work
is rich with solid referencing, crisply written narratives, and real-
life examples. Simply put, Drs. Moss and Shaw-McMinn have
delivered the new standard bearer for excellence in eyecare practice management.

My advice—tackle this book head on. Immersion in this work
will catalyze you to reinvent your approach to health care business, and of course, don't forget to enjoy reaping the rewards.

*Barry J. Barresi, O.D., Ph.D.*

# Preface

Our intent in this book and additional texts to follow is to assist the eyecare professional (ECP) in developing the select skills and knowledge essential to succeed in today's marketplace. The health care environment has become quite challenging, requiring providers to accept and adapt to changes more rapidly and frequently than ever before. This need for continual monitoring is the result of ongoing events, causing the transformation of traditionally accepted models of eyecare delivery. A stable marketplace is predictable, offering few chances for creativity and breakthrough developments; today's relatively uncertain marketplace offers greater obstacles yet more opportunity to capable ECPs willing to accept the challenge. To compete effectively and achieve maximal goals and profitability, the ECP must be flexible, able to plan for and adapt to rapid change, and able to predict likely future events by recognizing and understanding recent trends affecting the ophthalmic industry. According to Bhatt Vadlamani, Ph.D., instructor in strategic management, developing strategy is "like navigating in the fog."[1] Given the rapid changes in health care reform, consolidation, oversupply of providers, dwindling resources, projected increase in consumer demand, increased regulatory and employee pressure, managed care certainly will continue to interject elements of uncertainty for the eyecare strategist throughout the first decade of the next millennium.

---

[1]Stated during lecture in a strategic management class of the MBA program at University of Massachusetts, Boston, summer 1996.

Our intent is to enhance the reader's understanding of influential forces in eyecare provider decision making. Our goal is to redirect discussions relevant to eyecare business from a traditional foundation based on anecdotal experience to a foundation rich in generally accepted business principles. This enhanced understanding is achieved through proven academic business theory supported by current research. These basic concepts should facilitate strategic business planning and implementation; "success in challenging times requires extraordinary commitments to operating efficiency, technology utilization, product quality and customer satisfaction."[2]

This text is directed toward the roles and tasks of the ophthalmic decision maker, whether it be as leader, owner, partner, or manager. The eyecare decision maker must possess a basic understanding and minimum level of competence in the six major disciplines affecting decision making: management, marketing, strategy development, communications, technology, and finance. These disciplines should be well understood to effectively direct personnel, promote a practice, and develop the necessary tactics to achieve desired business objectives.

When developing strategy in any business endeavor, future planning is based on assumptions made from recent industry trends and performance. The text will identify whenever such assumptions have been made. This text is not meant to be a complete, solitary resource on business theory but rather a discussion of concepts on specific topics to enhance your daily practice operations. As Johnson & Johnson CEO Ralph S. Larsen states: "Reputations reflect behavior you exhibit day in and day out through a hundred small things. The way you manage your reputation is by always thinking and trying to do the right thing everyday."[3]

Recent trends in health care delivery show that HMOs and managed care organizations are either losing profits or have been forced to increase premiums due to rising costs.[4] This trend will affect eyecare practice in the future in several different ways.

[2]Schermerhorn J. *Management*. New York: Wiley and Sons; 1999:4.
[3]*Fortune*. February 10, 1992:40–70.
[4]*Boston Globe*. July 29, 1999:D-1.

First, patient benefits, offered by employers, may become a defined contribution in partial payment toward the employee's health plan at an amount substantially reduced from their present levels or, in some cases, eliminated entirely. Reimbursement for existing services will either remain constant or possibly decrease. Additional mergers and consolidations within the managed care industry may result in fewer, larger managed care organizations.

Each chapter includes an action plan that reiterates what we believe are standards of performance that should be developed by each ECP who endeavors to create a strategic marketing plan for his or her eyecare business. Chapter 1 describes several fundamental components of a marketing program based on the needs of contemporary eyecare practice. Chapters 2, 3, 4, and 6 build on an understanding of the components necessary to create a marketing plan for the ECP's particular situation. Chapter 8 focuses on marketing high-quality service and the components of quality ECPs should consider when creating a marketing program for eyecare settings.

The concept of "moment of truth" analysis is elaborated on in Chapter 5, dealing with building long-term patient relationships, while "service blueprinting" is explained in Chapter 9, on implementing strategy. These are methods of identifying crucial interaction points between patients and ECP staff members that greatly influence the patient's perception of quality in the office. Many studies have been undertaken to determine what providers can do to enhance the value patients receive during office encounters. The effect of high-quality service delivery on patient satisfaction is examined in Chapter 7, because high-quality care is not synonymous with patient satisfaction and does not always translate into increased revenue or patient loyalty, both essential ingredients of practice longevity. Finally, Chapter 10 describes new marketing technology, using the Internet, that offers ECPs first-mover competitive advantages; and Chapter 11 covers marketing a practice for sale or purchase.

*G.L.M.*
*P.G.S-M.*

# Acknowledgments

I would like to acknowledge the following people and organizations for their various contributions to this book: Cindy Hutchison, Claire Rork, Marc McGee, and Marek Jacisin of the New England College of Optometry Library. They were instrumental in supplying me with hard-to-find electronic journal articles in a timely fashion, and in making the Library such a wonderful, cutting-edge resource with a great atmosphere in which to work. Laura Cochrane for the vast amount of downloading and typing she did for me, and Nikki Slagle for the fine job of refining and editing my initial thoughts and phrases. The Kirstein Branch of the Boston Public Library, possibly the finest, most complete business materials resource in the world. Christine Bell of the Newton-Wellesley Hospital Library for supplying specific, current healthcare business journals. Audrey Ashton-Savage and Ellen Bentoudja of Emmanuel College for giving me the opportunity to practice and refine my own knowledge base. My coauthor, Peter G. Shaw-McMinn for contributing the portions that filled in the voids, making this book practical and relevant for practicing ECPs. The American Optometric Association for developing the Practice Enhancement Program Monograph Series and The Association of Practice Management Educators for setting the high standard that we strive to achieve.

I would like to thank Master Un Hak Jung of Alpha Tae Kwon Academy for helping me find the internal energy, and my wife Traudi, and daughters Amber and Blaise, for providing the external motivation I needed to complete this project. I can't forget my mother Eva, sister Jamie, and nephews Hunter and Tanner. Finally, I dedicate this book to the memory of my father, Herbert L. Moss of Woodbridge, NJ, a pioneering breed of optometrist that will soon become just a memory to our profession.

*G.L.M.*

Gary has acknowledged many of the individuals that helped us write this book. In addition, I'd like to thank Dr. Richard L. Hopping, who has been a mentor to me and oversaw the development of The American Optometric Association Practice Enhancement Programs; Dr. John Larcabal for the support and marketing ideas he has provided us; Dr. Craig Hisaka for constant reminders of the humanistic side of marketing; the many doctors who contributed quotes to this book; and most of all, thanks to Gary L. Moss himself, for keeping on me about completing this book together and giving me the opportunity to contribute.

I'd like to acknowledge the tens of thousands of eyecare practitioners all over North America who have dedicated their lives to patient care and contributed to the positive images of the eyecare industry. Sometimes we forget who our competition is. The consumer has many different services and products asking for their time and money. Marketing is communicating, and who is better at communicating what we have to offer than the eyecare practitioner who effectively communicates the benefits of our services, improving the lives of our patients while enhancing the entire eyecare industry. We acknowledge the past efforts of these individuals who have made marketing and the opportunity to be successful easier for all of us. Thank you.

*P.G.S-M.*

# EYECARE BUSINESS

# CHAPTER 1

# Creating Your Practice Identity

The road to success is always under construction.
                                                    —*Lily Tomlin*

## Why Do You Need to Market?

Marketing as a distinct function occupies a position of prominence in the business plan of many eyecare offices. According to the U.S. Bureau of the Census,[1] nearly one third of American households relocate annually, adding to the challenge for the eyecare professional (ECP) to retain patients. For your practice to remain a high priority to patients, an ongoing communication program is necessary to strengthen your identity and to avoid becoming the community's "best kept secret." A well-crafted marketing program can enhance practice revenue growth, provide greater future benefits, and act as an annuity by increasing practice value. **ECPs compete against other industries for diminishing consumer dollars. The better we position the business and image of eyecare professionals in our society, the more secure the eyecare profession becomes and the stronger our ability is to endure downturns in the economy.**

In most communities, ECP offices are not overwhelmed by competition from other providers. However, ECPs consistently are confronted with the challenge to increase patient volume or local market share while attempting to decrease expenses and use fewer resources. Traditional advertising goals aim to create awareness of one's practice within the community and encourage patients to return for regular care. **Today's ECP must use effective,**

1

measurable, and well-targeted marketing tactics. Without a properly implemented business strategy, a practice may encounter flat revenues, decreasing market share, minimal growth of new patients, and loss of retained patients using the office.

Why does an ECP need to market at all? Many patients quickly forget about their ECP and many move to a location that is less convenient, making them less apt to return to your office. It is estimated consumers receive over 2,000 marketing messages per week through a variety of media.[2] Because of this bombardment of media communications, your marketing must be continual, iterative, and focused to maintain patient loyalty. Despite the vast penetration of managed care in creating a patient base, many ECPs mistakenly assume that managed care plans drive patients into their offices. Potential problems may occur for the ECP who willingly delegates the marketing responsibility to a third party. Patients and insurance programs are in a constant state of flux, often changing annually, either through a change in benefits or change in health plans offered by employers. This creates a great deal of uncertainty for the ECP planning business strategies and making revenue projections. However, by taking the time to develop specific marketing goals and programs, you can find opportunities within the changing health care marketplace.

The primary goal of marketing is to obtain, retain, and educate patients by creating a practice image that embodies the trust you develop with your patients. The processes by which this goal can be achieved are:[3]

- Develop a strategy that emphasizes the unique features your practice offers.
- Educate patients to influence their purchase decision making.
- Identify patients most likely to value your services and to respond to your marketing.
- Position your products and services favorably in your local community.

Each of these requirements presents different challenges to influence patient spending patterns while matching practice sales tactics to current local marketplace conditions. The ECP responsible for marketing an eyecare business must preserve a consistent image focused on patient needs and wants reinforced by the entire staff's actions.[4]

## Developing a Strategy

The key to addressing changes in today's eyecare market is flexibility. Consider basing your strategic marketing decisions on the following criteria:

1. Differentiate your products and services while emphasizing your unique attractiveness to potential patients.
2. Select and use the most advantageous promotional methods to deliver your message.
3. Apply a cost-effective criteria to the selection of marketing tactics while projecting and justifying profitability.
4. Base your marketing decisions on resources and capabilities available to you.
5. Take into account the perceived benefits that patients value and how these will produce desired patient satisfaction, continued loyalty, and referrals.

Once developed, the marketing plan offers the roadmap for you to follow. The following six areas are primary components of marketing strategy that require critical decision making when action is taken by the ECP:[5]

1. Evaluate patient needs and identify areas where the ECP can create value.
2. Identify specific segments of patients to whom you wish to market your services.
3. Determine all the people in a position to refer new patients and the various methods available to distribute your marketing message.
4. Analyze the quality, readiness, and ability of your communications program to deliver your marketing messages.
5. Determine the image you wish to convey and develop marketing tactics that convey the unique benefits your practice offers.

6. Assess the effectiveness and untapped potential of the in-office point-of-purchase materials.

## Influencing Patient Purchasing Decisions

To have a greater impact on the outcome, an eyecare provider should have a complete understanding of the various components and stages of the patient purchasing process, which can be divided into the six stages shown in Table 1–1.[3] The patient starts the process when the decision is made to purchase eyecare. The response that the ECP ultimately makes can influence the patient's final purchasing decision. Directing each facet of the overall patient purchasing process on a proactive basis prevents patient attrition or a decrease in community awareness of your practice's capabilities.

How can the ECP influence this process and possibly "change" a patient's behavior, attitude, or belief? "Inducing a

**Table 1–1    Stages in the Purchasing Process: Patient Event and ECP Actions**

| | |
|---|---|
| Step 1. | Patient event: The patient must recognize the need for eyecare or an office visit.<br>ECP action: Generate patient awareness or need via some media channel, such as public relations, mailings, or recall. |
| Step 2. | Patient event: The patient recalls information or prior sources of satisfaction that can be transferred to use with the present need.<br>ECP action: Reinforce or associate need with available brands and health plans in which ECP participates. |
| Step 3. | Patient event: The patient evaluates all alternatives available.<br>ECP action: Influence with informative supporting materials (pull strategy). |
| Step 4. | Patient event: The patient applies personal criteria and makes any necessary compromises due to changes in personal situation or limited availability.<br>ECP action: Offer opinions and advice (push strategy). |
| Step 5. | Patient event: The patient makes a choice.<br>ECP action: Dissipate any lingering obstacles. |
| Step 6. | Patient event: The patient does a postpurchase analysis.<br>ECP action: Minimize cognitive dissonance or any lingering doubt. |

change in behavior is called compliance. Inducing a change in attitude is called persuasion. Inducing a change in belief is called either education or propaganda—depending on your perspective."[6] According to Drs. Kelton Rhoads, Ph.D., and Robert Cialdini, Ph.D., there are six principles an ECP can employ in his or her marketing tactics: consistency, reciprocation, social proof, authority, liking, and scarcity.[7] One technique that enhances provider ability to persuade patients used by Art Kobayashi, O.D., of Wahiawa, Hawaii, is: "I learned how to steer the conversation while listening."[8]

To be effective, point of purchase strategies require that your employees understand, accept, and support your marketing plan. Make sure employees possess the skills and training needed to correctly supply requests for information or the results of any planned marketing strategy will be compromised at the onset. Your current practice management information system software must be adequate to handle the capacity necessary to achieve the goals of your marketing program. **Employee behavior and system resources should optimize marketing effectiveness.**

## Identifying Which Patients to Reach

Meeting expectations is fundamental to achieving patient satisfaction, which creates perceived value; begin the patients' needs assessment by asking what products and services patients need and value. Obtaining patient opinions may help identify new marketing opportunities. Once this is decided, determine how you can maximize the effectiveness of your marketing to address the patient needs so identified and motivate a response.

The effectiveness of a marketing strategy is the result of how you develop and distribute your marketing message through the various media available to you and how you emphasize the benefits and features that set you apart from your competition.[9] This will determine the position you occupy in your particular market. The media you choose should generate awareness of your services and result in patient inquiries and appointments. If you choose mass media advertising, it must be consistent and frequent. Simple, small ads appearing often in targeted publications are more effective than large, infrequent ads appearing in wide-spread circulation.[9] Finally, you must select the marketing tools, method of distribution, and budget allocation you will use to deliver your marketing message. **Recognize what features are desired by patients and exploit the benefits offered by these features in your office marketing program.**

Targeted market identification involves dividing the local population into patient groups most likely to use the services of your practice. This strategy, referred to as *segmentation*, increases the return on your marketing outlay while decreasing the cost to acquire new patients. Segmentation offers a higher return than mass marketing and focuses on specific groups while attempting to directly influence their purchasing decisions. Chapter 4 discusses in detail the segmentation process as it applies to eyecare practice. Examining present marketing tactics and planning for future changes and improvements will help you target and reach the most favorable patient groups. **Identify and reach those groups with the highest likelihood of utilizing your services.**

## Positioning Your Practice

Of prime importance is to coordinate the delivery of the final communications message, broken down into six steps:

1. Decide how you want your marketing message to appeal to your patients.
2. Choose the content of your marketing message.
3. Select the method to distribute your marketing message.
4. Ascertain what resources are required to convey your marketing message.
5. Determine the budget available for marketing.
6. Anticipate what response, if any, your competitors may make to your marketing initiative.

To convey your desired marketing message, determine the "influencers" you believe you can use most effectively. These are the people, businesses, and means you may select to distribute your marketing message to patients. Commonly used people are primary care physicians, school nurses and athletic coaches, employee benefits managers, physician assistants, and welfare and social workers. Direct mail, print media, a website, and e-mail can be used to influence the appeal and effectiveness of your marketing message. **Recognize new and extraordinary means to convey your marketing message to direct patients to your services.**

Patients will perceive and retain your marketing message based on their needs. A patient's attitude is his or her point of view about the products and services you offer, while belief, which can influence a patient's attitude, involves the opinion he or she has formed.[10] Patient beliefs may significantly affect the final impact of the marketing messages you select and the channels you use to distribute the messages.[11] Channels are the various media or routes available to deliver your message. Mass media encompasses a widespread message delivered by newspaper or radio, while direct mail makes use of a much narrower route often generated by an in-office database of patient names and profiles.

Reinforcing a favorable attitude involves a decision to take some type of action, as in choosing a specific ECP. **Patient education through the marketing message can change a patient's attitude about a particular product or service, resulting in favorable response toward your practice.** Through an understanding of how patients obtain and retain information, you can exert positive influence on patient purchasing. One internal marketing opportunity an ECP has to influence patient perceptions is the professional biographies given to patients in the office. Appendix 1–1 offers an exercise in writing such a bio and Figure 1–1 shows a sample.

Research supports the claim that the majority of consumer behavior is learned.[12] You have an opportunity to exert a positive influence in the area of patient education. When you first introduce a new product or service, the focus should be on educating potential purchasers by emphasizing patient awareness. The ECP must *inform* patients about the benefits and advantages of the new product over current products and overcome any lingering purchasing obstacles. Direct mail and education of referral sources,

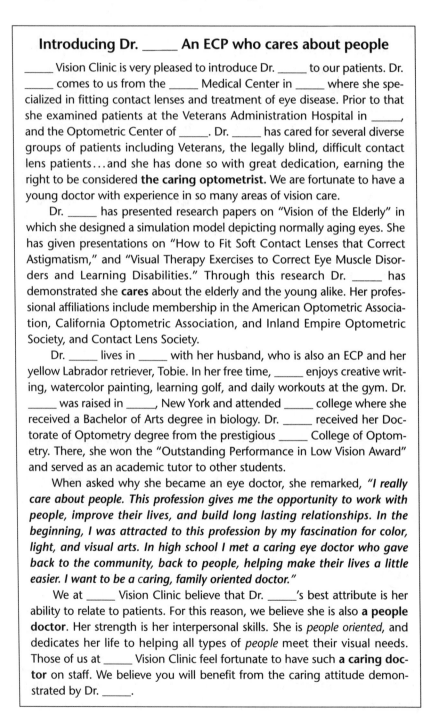

**Introducing Dr. _____ An ECP who cares about people**

_____ Vision Clinic is very pleased to introduce Dr. _____ to our patients. Dr. _____ comes to us from the _____ Medical Center in _____ where she specialized in fitting contact lenses and treatment of eye disease. Prior to that she examined patients at the Veterans Administration Hospital in _____, and the Optometric Center of _____. Dr. _____ has cared for several diverse groups of patients including Veterans, the legally blind, difficult contact lens patients…and she has done so with great dedication, earning the right to be considered **the caring optometrist.** We are fortunate to have a young doctor with experience in so many areas of vision care.

Dr. _____ has presented research papers on "Vision of the Elderly" in which she designed a simulation model depicting normally aging eyes. She has given presentations on "How to Fit Soft Contact Lenses that Correct Astigmatism," and "Visual Therapy Exercises to Correct Eye Muscle Disorders and Learning Disabilities." Through this research Dr. _____ has demonstrated she **cares** about the elderly and the young alike. Her professional affiliations include membership in the American Optometric Association, California Optometric Association, and Inland Empire Optometric Society, and Contact Lens Society.

Dr. _____ lives in _____ with her husband, who is also an ECP and her yellow Labrador retriever, Tobie. In her free time, _____ enjoys creative writing, watercolor painting, learning golf, and daily workouts at the gym. Dr. _____ was raised in _____, New York and attended _____ college where she received a Bachelor of Arts degree in biology. Dr. _____ received her Doctorate of Optometry degree from the prestigious _____ College of Optometry. There, she won the "Outstanding Performance in Low Vision Award" and served as an academic tutor to other students.

When asked why she became an eye doctor, she remarked, *"I really care about people. This profession gives me the opportunity to work with people, improve their lives, and build long lasting relationships. In the beginning, I was attracted to this profession by my fascination for color, light, and visual arts. In high school I met a caring eye doctor who gave back to the community, back to people, helping make their lives a little easier. I want to be a caring, family oriented doctor."*

We at _____ Vision Clinic believe that Dr. _____'s best attribute is her ability to relate to patients. For this reason, we believe she is also **a people doctor.** Her strength is her interpersonal skills. She is *people oriented,* and dedicates her life to helping all types of *people* meet their visual needs. Those of us at _____ Vision Clinic feel fortunate to have such **a caring doctor** on staff. We believe you will benefit from the caring attitude demonstrated by Dr. _____.

**Figure 1–1   Sample ECP office bio.**

such as primary care physicians, are two excellent and cost-efficient means to create initial patient interest. At the onset, prices can be higher because patients who are interested in the product often are motivated by "being the first to have it" and may not be as concerned with price. During this initial period, sales volume may be low, technical problems may arise, and costs may be high relative to revenue generated—these factors can be used to justify a higher price to the patient. The primary goal for the ECP is to create patient demand for the product or service being introduced. Once the product or service is introduced and accepted, patients may "become more discriminating and sophisticated in their purchasing behavior and product-use patterns."[13] At this juncture, a primary objective for the ECP is to increase market share and *persuade* more patients to choose the product or service through increased recognition. This is an excellent opportunity to take advantage of point-of-purchase materials obtained from vendors. ECPs who assume the risk of being the first to offer a new product or service usually benefit the most during this phase of greater demand. Caution should be exercised to prevent overspending or committing practice resources during this phase, because it is easy to be misled by a higher than normal demand, which will not last forever.

After the product or service is established, increased competition may force you to take measures to prevent patients from switching to other eyecare outlets. Typically, as demand begins to stabilize and revenues level off, any increase in market share often is at the expense of the competition rather than from a surge of new consumers entering the market. Price competition begins and advertising expenses can increase as a result, forcing the ECP to watch expenses even closer. An example of this life cycle of a product recently witnessed by many of us involves laser refractive surgery. **The goal for the ECP's marketing message is to differentiate your products and services by emphasizing the unique value you offer compared to your competitors.**

Once demand for a product or service has stabilized, the goal for the successful ECP is to maintain patient volume and prevent loss. Often, this will be achieved by demonstrating a distinct strategy in price, service, or promotional effort compared to the competition. The marketing goal is to *remind* patients to maintain their loyalty. Smaller practices may have found a core group of patients with which they have been successful. At this point, newer, unfamiliar, and superior products may become available to replace existing products that the ECP and staff are comfortable recommending and using. The ability to relinquish an existing commitment to established practice regimens and accept new patterns of business becomes a critical component of your marketing success.

Volume and revenue for a specific product variation eventually decreases, as patient demand is satiated and levels off. This gives you the choice of discontinuing, replacing, extending, or restarting a product or service. If a technologically superior product has been introduced, replacing the original product probably is the best route to follow. An example of this is radial keratotomy replaced by LASIK. Because both sales and market share typically have declined at this point, the ECP who decides to continue using the older version will have to *defend* his or her decision and point out to patients what advantages a particular product or service offers that individual. Figure 1–2 shows the relationship various marketing goals have relative to patient demand given the duration that a practice offers a particular product or service.

A variety of vehicles are available to deliver your message, including communications media, direct mail newsletters and brochures, brands and logos, alliances and networks, point-of-sale awareness materials, screenings, public addresses, newspaper columns, and co-op advertising. Be conscious of the inherent obstacles established by managed care to exploit uniqueness. While it can be argued that managed care lowers marketing costs for many health care practices, it often inhibits the ability to emphasize uniqueness by imposing limited benefits and standardized service or product offerings. **First, determine the most cost-effective strategies to generate patients and sales. Second, optimize your practice's competitive advantage by enhancing your uniqueness.** Remember that "in the minds of customers, frequency of valued contact equates to high loyalty in the relationship."[14]

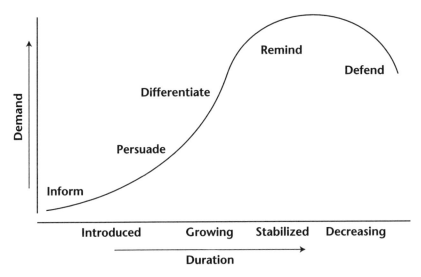

**Figure 1–2** Match your marketing message with patient demand. The vertical axis shows the annual percentage change in revenue as a function of the length of time a product or service has been offered. The figure shows that, during the introductory phase, as expected, there is little growth, but once the product or service is established, the revenue grows at a faster pace until leveling off during the mature phase.

## Creating Your Image Through Differentiation

A thorough assessment will uncover the best ways for you to use differentiation strategy in your marketing messages. Differentiation strategy consists of the various methods you choose to show patients how your products and services are unique and offer greater value than those of your competitors. Understanding the capabilities of your competitors will prove beneficial. For example, knowing whether your location offers a larger selection and greater variety of unique services than the competition is an advantage when developing your marketing program. Another situation to consider is how sufficient entry barriers prevent the likelihood of new arrivals threatening your existing market share. Observe the competition in your area and decide how to best differentiate your practice from theirs. Methods include a focus on technical expertise and specialty practice, innovations in product features and clinical testing procedures, appointment waiting time, lower costs and higher value, and expanded hours and number of locations.

Table 1–2 describes tactics that you can use to differentiate your business from the competition. One of these, extensions, uses the sale of complementary products to augment revenue. The alternative medicine industry has grown tremendously with consumers, approaching $21 billion dollars in annual sales. However, there is both opportunity for eyecare providers with the sale of nutraceuticals and also potential to abuse the claims being made about their benefits to patients. "Financial motives in medicine should never be primary. If they are, our core values are wrong. . . . If we are motivated by enhancing quality of care and

**Table 1–2    Differentiation Tactics to Use in a Marketing Program**

- *Extensions.*[a] Offer nontraditional products aimed at prevention. A list of companies and ocular products ECPs can offer their patients appears in the Appendix to the book.
- *Bundling.*[b] Combine various services or products into one integrated offering.
- *30-day call.*[c] Use this as both an informal survey tool and method to ascertain how satisfied the patient was with the service and is with any products purchased. The call also is useful to reduce any remaining cognitive dissonance patients might experience.
- *Charity-related marketing.*[d] This occurs when you select a social cause, event, or organization with which to associate practice marketing efforts. Choose one that is well known and appreciated in your community or closely associated with eyecare.
- *Website.* Your website offers the opportunity to provide patients with new and timely information during the entire year, not just when they are in your office.
- *Database.* Databases should be developed with detailed patient information and characteristics that allow you to contact specific groups of similar patients to offer products and services relevant to their needs or personal characteristics.

[a]Beiting J. The ethics of supplemental sales. *Eyeworld*. January 1999:26–27,36.
[b]Ovans A. Make a bundle bundling. *Harvard Business Review*. November–December 1997;75(6):18–20.
[c]Hansen L. Keep the customer satisfied. *Marketing Tools*. June 1998:45–58.
[d]Reidy C. Malls sold on charity related marketing. *Boston Globe*. February 10, 1999:F1.

we do a good job, the financial rewards will follow."[15] Another differentiating tactic an ECP can use is to offer patient incentives when bundling existing products, as when discounts are offered to patients purchasing a new contact lens fitting. Also, an affiliation or small local network of health care providers, such as dentists and pharmacists, can be formed to co-advertise within each other's office by offering exclusive discounts. In words of Joe Vitale, "Find businesses who are already serving your market and create an alliance with them."[16] Mr. Vitale also suggests "to make your place of business fun to visit; a place where your customers can feel good."[16] One tactic rarely used by eyecare providers is marketing the benefits of infection control in your office.[17] Prominently display office aseptic and OSHA written materials for patient education, sterilize your hands in front of every patient before the exam, and have your assistant wipe down exam room surfaces in front of the patient.

Another excellent way an eyecare practice can differentiate itself is through the variety and types of benefits patients receive. The exercise in Appendix 1–2 analyzes present benefits and indicates areas for possible future expansion. Determine how you want patients to perceive your practice and what you want patients to associate with the product and services you offer, then emphasize these benefits in the marketing messages you send. This should originate from your practice's mission and, in turn, be conveyed through the values you uphold. Often, this can be accomplished through alliances, network affiliations, brand promotions, and the universal use of your logo in all print media. **Clearly identify the position you choose to occupy in your market and make patients comprehend the value your practice offers relative to your competitors.**

## Developing the Marketing Plan

Table 1–3 shows the sequence of steps taken when developing a marketing plan. A marketing plan should reflect the results of patient demand analysis. This measures high and low usage periods for specific products or services, knowledge of your

**Table 1–3   Steps in the Marketing Plan Process**

1. *Determine marketing goals and objectives* (Chapter 2). Use your practice mission statement for guidance.
2. *Analyze the marketplace* (Chapter 3). Assess your current situation and any barriers to achieving your objectives. Utilize market research, data, and tools.
3. *Identify marketing opportunities* (Chapter 4). Analyze segmentation, targeting, and positioning of your present and potential patients.
4. *Build long-term patient relationships* (Chapter 5). Examine brands and patient loyalty.
5. *Manage the marketing mix* (Chapter 6). Use the four-P model to gain a competitive advantage. Use new technologies to promote your practice (Chapter 10).
6. *Understand product and service characteristics that patients value* (Chapter 7).
7. *Formulate a marketing plan and business strategy* (Chapter 8).
8. *Implement a marketing plan* (Chapter 9). Develop benchmarks and controls.

competitors' capabilities and weaknesses, and action plan program calendars that reflect budgeting with cost-benefit justification.

A well-conceived marketing plan should answer the following:[18]

1. What is the current condition of my practice?
2. In which direction should I take my practice?
3. How do I start in the correct direction?
4. How will I know when I have reached my objectives?

Short-term planning usually encompasses less than 1 year; intermediate planning, 1 to 2 years; and long-range planning, longer than 3 years. With the rapid changes in eyecare delivery demanding the need for flexibility, it would not be prudent to budget funds for any specific course of action much beyond two years into the future without contingencies in place or a means to redirect your funds should the need arise. This is supported by the management research of Elliot Jacques.[19] Jacques believes that most people are capable of working within a three-month planning range with no problem, but this number drops off significantly when planning 1 year ahead and only one person in several million can manage to plan the span of a 20-year career. At a minimum, any business or marketing plan you develop should include the following information:[20]

1. *Business description summary.* Include your mission, form of organization, unique characteristics, overview of your purpose, and key elements of your strategy.
2. *Community analysis.* Describe the size of your market and include relevant demographics, economic outlook for your target market, per capita income, and growth rate.
3. *Analysis of the eyecare industry.* Include economic trends, recent regulatory changes with significant impact, significant regional variations, and projected risk areas requiring attention.
4. *Analysis of the competition.* Include the number and type of competing optometrists, ophthalmologists, and opticians; draw a map and pinpoint each within a 1- and 5-mile radius (include 10 miles if located in a rural area). Describe the effect competition might have on your practice and how you will overcome the competition.
5. *Marketing plans.* Describe internal and external marketing strategies—ways of promoting yourself, goods and services you plan to offer, how patients will find out about you, and what industry trends will affect your practice.
6. *Operations.* Describe the methods you presently use, vendors used to obtain supplies, staffing requirements, human resource systems, compensation methods, and recurring practice expenses. How do you deliver, bill, and collect payment for services and products. Compare this data to national averages for the industry. If this data is unobtainable, a guideline to use is: fixed costs 40–48% of gross revenue, variable costs 24–32% of gross revenue, and net profit 26–34% of gross revenue.
7. *Financial projections.* Describe by service sources of revenue and expenses, quarterly for first year and annually for next 2 years, describe anticipated capital needs and expenditures.

Once you have determined your goals and objectives, initiate the marketing plan by first describing the existing segments of patients presently served, their size and potential.

Next, identify untapped segments of patients, their size and potential. From this, decide if any new segments of the market are viable or should be developed through awareness and education. To be effective, you must understand the various levels in which competition occurs as a function of patient demand for specific products or services. This will benefit the planning process and offer insight that can be used to enlarge your competitive strategy in daily operations.

Most well-run business ventures follow a marketing plan as a guide to accomplish and monitor desired communications goals; it should be no different for an ECP's office to achieve success. Specific functions must be performed in any marketing program that require data analysis, market research, and strategy development. **After determining your plan of action from a list of alternatives, implement, monitor, and initiate control mechanisms to properly evaluate the program's effectiveness.**

The mission statement you develop as part of the overall strategic plan of your office describes the long-term vision you have for your office and how you can highlight the unique qualities you offer.[21] This roadmap provides direction and motivation to your entire staff. Applying the wisdom of management theorist Peter Drucker to the eyecare setting, a business is "defined by the want the customer satisfies when he buys a product or service. Satisfying the customer is the mission and purpose of every business."[22] The mission you develop should be challenging, motivational, and optimistic. Keep in mind that, without a marketing strategy, a practice basically is in a commoditylike business, where the only basis for choice is price, resulting in the default strategy becoming the low-cost provider.[23]

To create a successful practice, acquire the resources and obtain the necessary marketplace research for developing a successful marketing strategy. The uncertainty of today's health care marketplace demands that ECPs not only meet the business needs of their practice but acknowledge and provide for the public health needs of their community. The following chapters discuss various methods to achieve the development of a strategic marketing program for eyecare practice. The ECP who is patient while using careful and prudent planning will realize this goal. In addition to the sequence of the process, Table 1–3 identifies the chapter in this book that covers each step in developing a marketing plan. The goal is for you to gain the ability to develop your own marketing plan by the end of the text.

> Render more service for that which you are paid and you
> will soon be paid for more than you render.
> —*Napoleon Hill* [24]

## Action Plan for ECPs

1. Review the various elements that constitute a successful marketing plan.
2. Recognize how and at what significant junctures the ECP can positively influence the patient purchasing decision.
3. Complete the exercises found in Appendix 1–1, Developing a Professional Bio, and Appendix 1–2, Differentiating an Eyecare Practice by the Benefits Provided, to determine what tactics you presently use to make your practice unique while enhancing the benefits patients receive.
4. Identify the stage of the life cycle of each product or service you want to promote and the type of message that would be most effective.
5. Consider and investigate the possible messages, media, and means available to achieve your marketing objectives.
6. Complete Assessing Your Marketing Effectiveness, Appendix 1–3, to become aware of the strengths and weaknesses in your marketing attitude before reading further. On completion, refer to page 23 for scoring and interpretation.

# Developing a Professional Bio

A patient will be more apt to agree with your recommendations if he or she trusts you as a doctor. One of the ways for a patient to learn about a doctor's qualifications is by reading a biographical sketch. Often the patient can learn something about you that facilitates the patient-doctor bond. For example, attending the same college provides a common link between your lives. Reading a biographical sketch prior to the first patient-doctor encounter can enhance the patient's opinion even before meeting you. The following is an outline for completing your biographical sketch.

1. *Title line.* "Introducing Dr. _____ . . ." [followed by brief description of what you stand for.] This is best chosen after you've completed the rest of the sketch.
2. *Paragraph on past clinical experience.* This can include outreach clinics you have been to or positions you have held in the past. It is best to mention the city and state where the clinic was located. This increases the chance the patient can relate to a geographical area.
3. *Research performed, speeches and papers written.* This statement gives you an opportunity to mention your expertise in an area that may be of interest to the patient.
4. *Professional affiliations.* Organizations to which you have membership, such as American Optometric Association, American Academy of Optometry or Ophthalmology, Optician Association of America.
5. *Community involvement.* Volunteer positions or membership in community groups.
6. *Personal life.* Tell where you were raised, went to high school, college. What your personal interests and hobbies are. Tell about your family.

7. *Reason for being in the eyecare profession.* Here is the most effective part of the sketch. This paragraph explains what you stand for. It tells the patient what you want to do for them. Include a direct quote. Often, this quote is printed in bold type for emphasis. If the patient reads nothing else, you want them to read this. This section will also help you decide on a few words describing your identity in the title above. Examples are "Dr. Smith, . . ." "an old-fashioned country doctor," . . . "the communicating doctor," . . . "the rehabilitative doctor," . . . "the dedicated doctor," . . . "the caring doctor," . . . "the best optometrist." Completing this exercise will show where you may need to brush up on your qualifications. Review the example in Figure 1–1. Use your biographical sketch with patients before you see them. You will find them saying how impressed they are with your qualifications. Other patients may ask about your golf game or children or where you grew up. In any case a professional bio will create a favorable impression before you meet them.

# Differentiating an Eyecare Practice by the Benefits Provided

1. List every benefit an office can provide to their patients.
2. Put an asterisk in front of the benefits your office can provide.
3. Rank these benefits in importance to the typical patient in your community by placing a number next to the benefit.
4. Identify benefits you do not presently provide but may consider.
5. Add to the list benefits not already identified.

A sample list follows:

Optician has ____ years' experience.
Free consultations
Located on a main street
Children's waiting area
Foreign languages spoken
Website and e-mail access
Doctor practicing for ____ years
Doctor teaches at _____
Special offers
Courtesy insurance billing for patients
Acceptance of insurance payments
Guarantee on frames for at least 1 year
Information packet of available services
Full-range eyewear
Provides every type of contact lens
Payment by credit card
45-minute examination
Free adjustments on glasses
Free polishing of contact lens
Recall on annual basis

In-office lab
Late hours
Saturday hours
Easy parking
Easy access for handicapped
Orthoptist, optician, O.D., M.D.
Free pickup of patients
Toll-free (800) phone number
Friendly staff
Full services, including
  Contact lens fitting
  Eye muscle exercises
  Low-vision aids
  Disease detection
  Disease treatment with medication
  Laser refractive surgery
  High-fashion frames
  Learning-related vision therapy
  Cataract surgery
  Retinal surgery

# Assessing Your Marketing Effectiveness[25]

Complete each sentence with the choice that is closest to your present situation.

1. I use a variety of marketing tactics and offer various ophthalmic products and services to different patient groups.
   a. Never
   b. On occasion
   c. Frequently
2. I introduce new products and services into my practice based on _____
   a. The need or when business is slow.
   b. The arrival of salespeople who show me what is new or selling well.
   c. Quick action and the opportunity to gain first mover advantage.
3. I know the likelihood of different patient groups that would use my office from the identification of segments and geographic drawing areas.
   a. Never
   b. Moderately well
   c. Very well
4. When I make business projections, I account for patient trends, changes in technology, changes in the local economy, new products, and anticipated health reform.
   a. No, I direct my effort on my personal and present patients' needs.
   b. Occasionally, I plan for the long term but the majority is concerned with only this year.
   c. I monitor both short- and long-term opportunities and threats that appear from changes in the marketplace.

5. Market research data and demographics about my area _____
   a. Are never obtained.
   b. Are obtained on an as-needed basis for specific marketing programs.
   c. Are obtained and monitored on a continual basis to assess changes in the marketplace of which I could take advantage.
6. When developing marketing plans, I involve staff, suppliers, and media salespeople.
   a. No, I rely on my own ideas.
   b. Occasionally, I ask someone's opinion about my plans or I let others develop the marketing and I have final approval.
   c. I make decisions only after much input and agreement among all concerned.
7. My current marketing strategy is _____
   a. Nonexistent or at best ideas previously tried by others.
   b. The same long-standing strategy I have used for years.
   c. A well-defined, changing, creative plan supported by market research and feedback.
8. Formal market planning at my office _____
   a. Occurs only when income or patient volume is down.
   b. Is good for occasional short intervals of 6 months or less.
   c. Is comprehensive and takes into account both short- and long-term goals.
9. I monitor the cost effectiveness and results of different marketing programs I use.
   a. Rarely, usually deciding to market by chance or out of desperation.
   b. Occasionally, if I believe something works well, I simply repeat it.
   c. Often, I track specific results and watch which programs work the best.
10. I use available resources as effectively as possible when developing marketing programs.
    a. Rarely, I am not even aware of all resources available to me.
    b. Occasionally, I am aware of some resources but do not take advantage of more than a handful, usually the same ones.
    c. Most of the time, I take complete advantage of all known existing resources and always seek out new sources.

Score your marketing effectiveness self-assessment as follows. The possible range is from 10 to 30, give yourself points for each response: A = 1 point; B = 2 points; C = 3 points.

Here is the interpretation:

10–14　Weak, present marketing attempts seem to be ineffective.

15–19　Fair, you have the awareness and motivation but need to modify your strategy.

20–25　Good, a bit more effort should provide desired result.

26–30　Excellent, you should be happy with the present results.

## Notes

1. U.S. Bureau of the Census, 1998.
2. Witkin G. Effective use of retail marketing database. *Direct Marketing*. December 1995;58(8):32–36.
3. Modified from Deutsch B. Charting a course with strategic marketing. *Bank Marketing*. September 1998;30(9):28–34.
4. McKay E. *The Marketing Mystique*. New York: AMACOM Publishers; 1998.
5. Suggested by Gombeski W. Better marketing through a principles-based model. *Marketing Health Services*. Fall 1998; 18(3):43–48.
6. Rhoades K, Cialdini R. The secret power of persuasion. *Dental-Town Magazine*. September 2000:8–10.
7. Cialdini R. *Influence the Psychology of Persuasion*. Quill Publishing; 1993.
8. E-mail, Survey of successful marketing tactics, July 25, 2000.
9. Trellis A. The 3Ms of marketing. *Builder*. February 1998; 21(2):192.
10. Perrault, W Jr, McCarthy, E. *Basic Marketing*. Boston: Irwin McGraw-Hill; 1999:160.
11. Fitzsimons G, Morwitz V. The effect of measuring intent on brand-level purchase behavior. *Journal of Consumer Research*. June 1996:1–11. Garbarino E, Edell J. Cognitive effort, affect and choice. *Journal of Consumer Research*. September 1997: 147–158.
12. For further discussion of consumer learning, see Gregan-Paxton J, John D. Consumer learning by analogy. *Journal of Consumer Research*. December 1997:266–284. Kim J, Lim J, Bhargava M. The role of affect in attitude formation. *Journal of the Academy of Marketing Science*. Spring 1998:143–152.
13. Corey R. Marketing strategy—an overview. Harvard Business School case no. 9-579-054.
14. Hansen L. Keep the customer satisfied. *Marketing Tools*. June 1998:45.
15. Gleser R. Getting rich isn't easy or the point. *MGMA Journal*. September–October 1999:43.
16. Vitale J. *There's a Customer Born Every Minute*. New York: Amacom; 1998.

17. Roth K. Marketing infection control. *Dental Economics*. June 1996:60–62.
18. Freitag A. PR planning primer. *Public Relations Quarterly*. Spring 1998:14–17.
19. Kiechel W. How executives think. *Fortune*. December 21, 1987:139–144.
20. Timmons J. *New Venture Creation*. Boston: Irwin Publishers; 1994:355.
21. Modified from a quotation in Shonberger R, Knod E Jr. *Operations Management: Serving the Customer*. Plano, TX: Business Publications; 1988:4.
22. Drucker P. *Management: Tasks, responsibilities, practices*. New York: Harper and Row; 1974:79.
23. Kotler P. From sales obsession to marketing effectiveness. *Harvard Business Review*. November–December 1977:67–75.
24. Greiner D, Kinni T. 1001 Ways to Keep Customers Coming Back. Rocklin, CA: Prima Publishing; 1999:29.
25. Modified from Kotler P. From sales obsession to marketing effectiveness. *Harvard Business Review*. November–December 1977:67–75.

# CHAPTER 2

# Marketing Goals and Objectives

Give me a stock clerk with a goal, and I will give you a man
who will make history. Give me a man without a goal, and I
will give you a stock clerk.

—*J.C. Penney*

The goals of a marketing program are based on the vision, intent, and mission statement the ECP creates for the practice. Once you have established the future course you want your practice to take, you can create and strive to achieve specific objectives. The goals of your marketing program will direct your strategy to completion. An eyecare business's intent, mission, goals, and objectives, while all focused on achieving similar outcomes, are each developed differently.

According to Gary Hamel and C. K. Prahalad of the Harvard Business School, strategic intent occurs when a business leverages internal resources and capabilities to accomplish what appears to be unattainable goals in the competitive environment.[1] The intent of your practice is internally focused, reflecting your capabilities and how resources and unique competencies will produce competitive advantages. Strategic intent forms the principles and assumptions on which your practice's strategic mission is created. The mission of your practice is externally focused, according to Michael Hitt of Texas A&M University, defining the purpose and scope of your operations in terms of the products and services offered and the prevailing current conditions in your affected marketplace.[2]

## The Practice Mission Statement

Mission statements are categorized as either strategic, defining the scope and marketplace position you want your business to occupy, or philosophical, describing the beliefs, values, and standards the business intends to uphold.[3] An abundant literature discusses the components of a mission statement. At a minimum, your practice mission statement should identify the patients you wish to serve, the patient needs you will satisfy, and how you intend to satisfy those needs.[4] However, studies show that many mission statements consist of broad generalizations rather than a singular pledge to uphold the intended values and beliefs of the business.[5]

When properly developed, the mission statement inspires individual practice uniqueness by describing the types of products and services you intend to offer, the patient groups you will serve, and how you plan to deliver your services to patients. Of primary importance, the mission should emphasize your beliefs about your patients, employees, and your local community.[6] A practice mission can provide direction, serve as a public relations tool, and guide your objectives to realize your long-term vision.[7] The mission statement, however, should not be defined so narrowly that it stifles attempts to reach full potential.[8] At a minimum, the mission statement should[9]

1. Be specific and able to influence employee behavior.
2. Center more on satisfying patient needs than on products and services.
3. Reflect the unique talents of your practice recognizing strengths and weaknesses.
4. Be flexible, identifying external marketplace opportunities and threats to your practice.

Baxter International, a $15 billion dollar health care company has a concise, well-stated mission:

> We will be the leading health care company by providing the best products and services for our customers around the world, consistently emphasizing innovation, operational excellence, and the highest quality in everything we do.

Baxter's strategy, which complements the mission, is "To effectively develop, empower, and motivate employees at all levels so that we all become totally dedicated to 'delighting' our customers."[10] These show a well-formulated health care-related mission statement and strategy. They are action oriented, displaying a central concern for the customer. They exploit the company's strengths, while recognizing the need to be flexible.

## Developing a Practice Mission Statement

The mission statement is the focus of your practice and a primary description of the ethical and business composite of your practice; it needs to be clear, unique, and focused. Those who read it should know immediately who you are and what you want to accomplish. Do you need a mission? One viewpoint was aptly expressed by former New York Yankees catcher and manager, Yogi Berra: "If you don't know where you are going in life you're liable to wind up someplace else." As the leader of your eyecare business you should "have a dream, a mission, and a strategic intent that is widely communicated, and has meaning to everyone in the organization."[11]

The questions in Table 2–1 will assist you in composing your mission statement. Consider your answers to these questions when deciding the patient needs your practice is most suited to address. Consider your resources, competitive position, and personal aspirations. Write generally how you intend to satisfy those

**Table 2–1  Questions to Ask in Developing a Mission Statement**

1. What is in it for me?
2. Why do I want to be an independent eyecare practitioner?
3. Who are my patients? Who should I add?
4. What values do my patients look for when they select my type of service?
5. Who are the other vision care providers in my area?
6. How am I different than the other ECPs in the area? How can I accentuate the difference?

Source: Modified from Your business and financial plan, Module 1. *AOA Practice Enhancement Program*, course workbook. St. Louis, MO: American Optometric Association; 1986:9.

patient needs. Ask yourself, How can I meet unsatisfied wants that may result from anticipated changes? What new satisfactions can I offer? What old, unproductive offerings can I abandon? How can I minimize my weaknesses?

Complete your mission statement and evaluate it using the exercise in Appendix 2–1. Write your final mission statement. Use it to guide your marketing decisions. All marketing should be consistent with your mission statement. If not consistent, you will lose credibility with your staff and patients. It is vital that all personnel accept your mission statement for your practice to be successful and credible to your patients.

An office meeting should be devoted to periodically review or revise the mission statement with staff input. Post the mission statement in areas around the office to remind the staff of your office representation. Utilize the mission statement as a marketing tool when communicating with patients. The following are several mission statements to use as examples while developing your own:

- Our mission is to build a practice in a three-county-area metropolis (population 40,000). The practice will provide technically advanced vision care services in an efficient manner to make these services affordable to the top 75% of the families in this area.
- Our mission is to build a practice in X-ville, an established community, to serve patients in the geographic area within 20 miles of X-ville to the north, 30 miles to the east, 50 miles to the south, and 30 miles to the west. The practice will provide convenient hours for the patients and the best level of service in this geographic area with a strong emphasis on sports vision.
- Our mission is to provide a practice in Woodcrest primarily serving 95% of the vision needs of all patients within 2 miles of the community. The practice will include opticians, optometrists, and ophthalmologists offering services in a patient-friendly manner with convenient hours, a comfortable office atmosphere, and payment plans for community members.

- Mission:
  To provide our patients and customers the highest level of
     eyecare services and products creating unchallenged
     loyalty, consumer satisfaction, and patient retention.
  To provide staff members a rewarding work environment,
     with the necessary resources, that offers opportunities
     for personal and career growth while recognizing any
     existing diversity.
  To be recognized by the community in which we are located
     as a caring, responsible business and concerned partner
     willing to perform volunteer services to those in need.
  To become a leader within the ophthalmic community by
     earning the respect of our colleagues through uncom-
     promised cooperation.
  To achieve maximum value and equity through the integra-
     tion of the latest technology with practice personnel
     and operations to gain all possible economic and finan-
     cial advantages.
  Motto—We make you *see* the difference!

## Practice Goals and Objectives

In Lewis Carroll's *Alice in Wonderland*, Alice asks the Cheshire Cat
which path to take, and he responds, "If you don't care where
you're going, it doesn't make a difference which path you take."
Without specific goals to achieve, you will tend to be more reactive than proactive. This is especially true when marketplace conditions offer an opportunity. It is much easier for an ECP to gain
competitive advantage when conditions are recognized to be
compatible with predetermined goals. Goals set the direction for
your strategies, whereas objectives signal the destination or the
desired result. Goals are open-ended; they're neither quantifiable
nor time limited. A single goal may have multiple objectives. Business objectives should be created using the SMART acronym to
make them proactive and geared toward successful completion:

Specific (fully describe in writing the desired results you want to
     achieve).

Measurable (objectives should be quantifiable, to monitor progress and for benchmark comparisons).

Achievable (determine what resources are needed and what resources you possess to achieve objectives).

Results oriented (objectives are outcomes, *not* just activities).

Time bound (objectives should have a defined time frame or milestone to achieve; when monitored, they can be revised if needed rather than continuing on endlessly).

Here is an example of business goals and their associated objective:

Goal: Increase contact lens revenues.

Objective: 10% increase in new fittings of contact lenses in 6 months.

Goal: Increase awareness of specialty services offered.

Objective: Increase number of new specialty vision training patients by 5% in 6 months. (Achieved by sending 1,000 direct mail newsletters within 4 months and writing 2 news articles for local newspaper within 3 months.)

Here are examples of various objectives, how they are measured, and their impact on the ECP's business:

*Practice Development*

Objective: Create a 1,200 patient database within 4 months.

Measure of success: Two mailings within 6 months of completing database.

Impact on practice: 10% increase in recall rate and updated database.

*Human Resource Development*

Objective: Initiate annual staff performance appraisal within 6 months

Measure of success: Feedback received from staff survey.

Impact on practice: Increase employee job satisfaction and patient services.

*Operations*

Objective: Eliminate excess capacity and underutilized income production.

Measure of success: 20% decrease in number of no-shows in 6 months.

Impact on practice: Increased revenues and more effective time management.

There are many areas of the ECP's business to which proper goal and objective assessment and development can be applied, as shown in Table 2–2.

Here is an example of a marketing communications goal:

Goal: Increase community awareness of the specialty services offered. (Examples chosen are vision training or low vision.)
Objectives:
1. Increase the number of new vision-training (VT) or low-vision (LV) patients by 10% within X months from today.
2. Send 2,000 direct mail newsletters to existing patients and/or 1,000 brochures to new patients describing VT or LV services within X months.
3. Write and have published two consumer news articles on either VT or LV for the local newspaper, the first within 2 months and the second no later than 6 months.

**Table 2–2   Business Objectives in an ECP's Practice**

| |
| --- |
| Increase net margins (profitability) |
| Decrease costs (efficiency and productivity) |
| Increase total revenue (growth and market share) |
| Improve resource utilization (return on both assets and investment) |
| Increase practice value (appreciation) |
| Demonstrate social responsibility (community involvement) |
| Enhance employee benefits (security and wages) |
| Apply technological innovations (reputation and image) |

4. Make a presentation about the benefits of VT to the local parent-teachers' association or LV to a local senior citizens' club.

These are examples of a marketing objective:

*Objective for Practice Development*
1. To create a 2,000 patient database using new practice management software within 6 months of today.
2. To measure the success of such efforts by completing two mailings within 3 months of completing the database.
3. The desired impact on the practice is that 15% of the patients will receive a mailing to contact the office for information generated from the mailing. Enhancement of the quality of future mailings by updating the database with returned change-of-address notices will be a high priority.

There are several reasons why you might not have goals: You don't know what you want, you don't believe goals will work, you confuse working hard with working smart, you don't understand the true function of goals, or you do the urgent instead of the important. Take the time to carefully craft and review your goals every 6 months. If marketplace conditions change, you may need to modify your goals and the strategy developed to achieve those goals.

Aim at nothing and you'll probably hit it.

—*Anonymous*

## How Goals Reflect Your Mission

To develop a mission statement reflecting the vision, intent, and mission for your office, you must first look to your personal and professional goals. Recognizing what you want in your personal and professional life will guide you toward a mission consistent with other aspects of your life. Often this is the most difficult step. Have you ever sat down and set goals for your life? Did you write them down? Most of us, if asked, would like a successful life. Being a success means different things to different people.

The actress Carol Burnett defines success as "getting a good seat in a restaurant, eating marvelous food, meeting an awful lot of nice people, being able to go to the dentist twice a year and being quoted in the magazines. Best of all, success means having enough closet space!" Garfield, our favorite cat, defines success as, "Being able to eat 20 pizzas without throwing up." How would you define success in your particular case? For this discussion, one way to simplify what is meant by *success* is to use this definition: Success is getting what you want.

Once you determine what you want, you will be able to measure your level of success. The first step in planning your mission for your office involves setting your personal goals. Although your goals are certain to change with time, it is easier to plan once you have an idea of the final destination. Many people might like to become a leader in their community. Others would like to be an acknowledged leader in their profession. A closer look at some simple facts will help you see how to start working in the upper percentile of successful people. The average person is out of school 4 years before he or she starts thinking about goals and, by that time, usually is married with one child. Less than 5% of the population set goals. Less than 1% of those who have goals write them down.[12] By setting goals and writing them down, you can become a member of an elite group of people who have a plan for success.

## Personal and Career Goals

Whether you are a recent graduate embarking on a new career, an established practitioner nearing retirement, or somewhere in between, the decisions you make affecting your personal and professional life will depend on what you want—your goals. Young graduates are concerned with paying off loans, buying a car, and perhaps purchasing their first home. Other goals may include traveling, perhaps joining the local country club, or constructing a new building for their practice.

The main resource recent graduates lack to reach these goals is money. Recognizing this need, the first decision to make related to professional practice is choosing a practice opportunity that provides this necessary resource, income. The recent graduate asks, "How can I get the money I need to get what I want and do what I want?" He or she initially may work for someone, then begin a practice of his or her own. What is your vision of the rest of your life? Where can you see yourself next year, 5 years, 10 years from now? What values are important to you? Answering these questions can require introspection. Psychologists use exercises to help guide people along the way. One such exercise to assist in developing personal goals that involves only a few minutes of time is shown in Appendix 2–2.

Completing this exercise truthfully will allow you to recognize what you value as important to you. Identifying your values will prepare you for setting personal and professional goals. Setting personal and professional goals will help you decide on the direction your practice must go; it guides you toward a mission statement.

When creating a mission statement, consider professional goals in addition to personal goals. Take a moment to visualize where ideally you will be 10 years from now. What practice situation will you be in? What is your role within your profession? How will you contribute to your community? What will your plans be for the third week in October, 1 year from today or 3 years from today? Appendix 2–3 is a survey form you can use in planning your professional goals for the future.

By focusing on personal and professional goals, the appropriate mission statement, marketing goals, and marketing objectives can be developed. Suppose your personal goals require more time out of the office. This need may require you to find an associate to continue providing the proper vision care in your absence. You could have Saturdays off to attend your children's soccer games, Wednesdays off to play golf, and perhaps squeeze a month of vacation time for cruises and other travel. Perhaps you want to give something back to your profession by joining the board of your local society and working your way up the chairs to state or national president. This takes time out of the office. Who will cover for you in the office?

## Why You Do Not Set Goals

What hinders people from setting goals? People do not set goals for four main reasons.[13] First, people don't understand the importance of goals. Research shows that goal setting and planning are the most important steps to success. Articles written in newspapers and magazines on a regular basis point out that success begins with goal setting. Leon A. Danco, CEO of The Center for Family Business, spent the past 35 years advising thousands of family-owned businesses. He explains, "Anybody who wants to be a success has got to think about the end before he gets engaged in the beginning. . . . You have to commit to the longevity of your business."[14] Setting goals does not end with an initial plan: "Unlike New Year's resolutions that are resolved once and never accomplished, our career and life's resolutions must be reviewed periodically. As we get older, our needs may change. We must evaluate our careers and ask ourselves if they are helping us achieve our long-term goals."[15] Long-term goals should be reviewed and revised on a yearly basis, due to rapid changes in the marketplace and regulatory rulings affecting eyecare practice. Staff members, friends, and family are valuable sources that should be included for feedback.

Second, people do not know how to set goals. In addition to being the most important step to success, goal setting is the most difficult step. Setting goals requires a process, a procedure, and a talent that is acquired through learning. Keep in mind you have set goals in the past, to some extent (to complete your college education, graduate, pass board examinations), and you succeeded. Ask yourself the following questions: What do I want to get out of my career? What is my vision for the future? How compatible are my personal goals with my professional goals? How compatible are my goals with my spouse's and family's goals?

The third reason people do not set goals is fear of rejection. Achieving goals often means making mistakes. Sometimes, you must try ideas to see what works best. You may be required to apply for a desired position ten times before you finally are accepted. You may have to prescribe certain treatments two or three different ways to a select group of patients before your advice stops being rejected. Fear of rejection is something you can control yourself. Nobody can control how you think. Use rejection as motivation for choosing a different strategy in achieving the goal.

The final reason for not setting goals is fear of failure; some people are fearful of never reaching their goal. It takes a level of confidence and bravery to declare a goal. Some think to themselves, "What will people think if I don't make it? What will they say when I fail?" Do you fear the possibility of being humiliated? Perseverance is one key to success in this area, in addition to a strong belief in your ideas. One positive way to approach fear of failure is summarized by a quote from football coach Lou Holtz: "If we succeed 100% of the time we are not trying hard enough. We are conservative. Failure is a normal fact of achievement."[16]

Success plans including goals actually produce less disappointment. As you focus on your goals, you will be able to monitor your progress. You gradually will become aware of the inability to reach a goal instead of suddenly feeling like a failure. Planning to reach goals actually prepares you for setbacks, so expect to gain a good understanding of why the goal was not reached. This leads to reevaluating future goals and strategies and to producing consistent results, quicker outcomes, and more accomplishments. Achieving the steps toward a major goal will motivate you toward trying harder. One example is losing weight. Weight loss is difficult to accomplish. But once you start to lose weight, become quicker on the tennis court and fit into clothes you haven't worn for years, this will motivate you to continue with enthusiasm. A sense of accomplishment can encourage you to pursue greater achievements.

Having goals allows you to measure your progress toward your mission. Goals are necessary in order to answer the question, "How's it going?" By beginning with your personal goals, you provide the best possible basis for building professional and career goals that allow you to develop a vision for your unique practice. Are your personal goals up-to-date? Do you need more time or money to reach your goals? The exercise in Appendix 2–4 will assist you in determining your future plans. The next time you decide what to do with your time or money, ask yourself, "How will this help me reach my goals?" Focus on these needs and develop a mission statement for your office that leads you to success.

## Developing Marketing Goals and Objectives

Use your mission statement to assist you in writing marketing goals and objectives for your practice. The following breaks the process into the necessary steps:

*Selection.* Brainstorm to create marketing goals and objectives consistent with your mission statement. Table 2–3 offers suggestions.

*Analysis.* Analyze these goals and set their priority based on factors such as
  a. What rewards come from successfully achieving this goal?
  b. How meaningful is this specific goal to my success plan?
  c. Am I convinced of the need for achieving this goal and willing to change habits and attitudes to accomplish it?
  d. Is it consistent with my personal, professional, and family goals?

*Support.* Build support systems for achieving the goal. What resources do you need to achieve it? Are financial, professional, personal, family, and community support available? Table 2–4 lists possible sources of assistance for the ECP.

*Feedback.* Establish feedback procedures and systems by which you can monitor how you are progressing toward the goal. Divide the goal into measurable events that show progress toward its achievement. Table 2–5 shows one method of monitoring progress.

*Imaging.* Visualize the accomplishment of the goal. Picture your goal in your mind and imagine its achievement. The mental image of a goal is the most motivating, powerful influence on reaching the goal. It helps you become motivated and shape your behavior in the right direction, to begin to break old habits and attitudes, and it triggers the energy needed to succeed. Visualization will keep you focused on your target. Carefully analyze it, build the support and feedback you

**Table 2–3  Choosing Marketing Goals**

| Statement | Yes | No | Maybe |
|---|---|---|---|
| 1. Increase the patient load | | | |
| 2. Improve patient satisfaction | | | |
| 3. Attract and keep new patients | | | |
| 4. Retain current patients | | | |
| 5. Increase income per patient | | | |
| 6. Become more financially secure | | | |
| 7. Become better known in the community | | | |
| 8. Become better known among health care professionals | | | |
| 9. Provide vision therapy services | | | |
| 10. Provide sports vision services | | | |
| 11. Co-manage laser refractive surgery | | | |
| 12. Provide low-vision services | | | |
| 13. Provide other services (specify) | | | |
| 14. Be recognized as a vision care spokesperson | | | |
| 15. Increase patient load for a new associate | | | |
| 16. Increase number of senior citizen patients | | | |
| 17. Increase number of contact lens patients | | | |
| 18. Increase populations of other patients | | | |
| 19. Increase number of referrals from educators | | | |
| 20. Decrease the amount of time spent on patient care | | | |
| 21. Provide care for low-income populations | | | |
| 22. Provide new ophthalmic products to patients | | | |
| 23. Sell contact lens solutions | | | |
| 24. Sell spectacle accessories to patients | | | |
| 25. Increase the number of multiple purchases of eyewear | | | |
| 26. Increase the number of patients seen from a specific part of the community | | | |
| 27. Increase the number of patients seen with annual incomes over $60,000 | | | |
| 28. Sell the practice within the next ___ years | | | |
| 29. Other (specify) | | | |

**Table 2–4    Marketing Resources for ECPs**

---

Staff
Legal assistance
Public relations person
Family
Professional association
Mentors
Community associations
Friends
Educators
Financial advisor
Colleagues
Other (specify)

---

**Table 2–5    Monitoring Goals**

---

Today's date:
    Specific goal:
    Specific benefits of reaching goal:
Target date:
    Where am I today with regard to the goal?
Obstacles to achievement?
Checkpoint dates:
    Intermediate Goal 1:
    Intermediate Goal 2:
    Intermediate Goal 3:
    Intermediate Goal 4:
Plans for surmounting obstacles:
Specific actions to take to form new habits:
Date goal was met:

---

need, and keep a clear mental focus on the goal. After completing your goals and objectives, the next step in a marketing plan is an analysis of your current situation. The process of analyzing goals and opportunities for the ECP is covered in the next chapter.

Developing marketing goals will serve many functions throughout the career of an ECP. The American Marketing Association has defined *marketing* as, "The process of planning and executing the conception, pricing, promotion, and distribution of goods and services to create exchanges that satisfy individual and organizational objectives."[17] Once you have developed your goals, you are in a better position to determine the marketplace opportunities most compatible with those goals. Methods you can use to identify marketplace opportunities are discussed in the next chapter.

## Action Plan for ECPs

1. Evaluate and modify your mission statement using Evaluating a Mission Statement (Appendix 2–1).
2. Complete Setting Personal Goals in Three Minutes exercise to recognize what values are important to you (Appendix 2–2).
3. Complete Setting Professional Goals exercise to demonstrate what direction your planning must take (Appendix 2–3).
4. Utilize Future Plans exercise to develop personal goals and objectives using the SMART acronym (Appendix 2–4).
5. Develop a business mission using questions from Table 2–1. Consider the various patient populations that come in contact with your practice, how you affect them, and how they affect you.
6. Chose marketing goals and objectives from Table 2–3.
7. Identify the resources required to achieve your goals and objectives (see Table 2–4), what obstacles must be overcome, and what competencies must be acquired.

## APPENDIX 2–1

# Evaluating a Mission Statement[18]

1. How clear am I on what my practice is right now? I have _____
   a. No idea.
   b. A vague idea.
   c. A pretty good idea.
   d. The complete picture.
2. Is my perception of what my practice is right now based on how I see myself or how my patients see me?
   a. Based on how I see myself.
   b. Mostly based on how I see myself.
   c. Mostly based on how my patients see me.
   d. Based on how my patients see me.
3. To what extent have I integrated my mission statement into the day-to-day operations of my practice?
   a. Not at all.
   b. Not much.
   c. Largely integrated.
   d. Totally integrated.
4. How clear is my mission statement in describing what I wish my practice to become?
   a. Not clear.
   b. Somewhat clear.
   c. Fairly clear.
   d. Completely clear.
5. To what extent does my mission statement focus on what the patient is receiving rather than what I think I am giving?
   a. Describes skills provided by the eyecare practitioner.
   b. Describes mostly skills provided by eyecare practitioner.
   c. Mostly describes patients' needs.
   d. Describes patients' needs.

6. To what extent does my mission statement anticipate change?
   a. Based on present practice.
   b. Mostly based on present practice.
   c. Mostly anticipates change.
   d. Anticipates change.
7. What would make the mission statement better?

# APPENDIX 2–2

# Setting Personal Goals in Three Minutes[16]

1. For 1 minute, write down all the goals you have for the rest of your life. Everything you can imagine you want to have or want to do.
2. For the next minute, write down all the goals you can think of for the next 2 years.
3. During the final minute, assume the following scenario: You have been diagnosed with cancer. Your physician gives you 6 more months to live. What would be your goals during those 6 months?

The answer to the first question allows you to brainstorm on goals that may come immediately to your mind. They may prove to be important to you on further analysis, or they may not. It at least gives you an idea of what comes to mind.

The second question forces you to look at goal setting within a time frame. Time is an important part of any goal. The answer to this question may indicate that these goals are more important to you. The answer to the third question often is quite different from the other two. The answers to the first two questions often include buying a Mercedes Benz, moving into a new house, being a community leader.

The answers to the third question commonly are spending more time with the family, traveling with the family, contributing effort to your church, doing more things with your friends. One way of putting it is that the goals change from "things" to "people." This may or may not be true in your case. Nevertheless, completing this exercise truthfully allows you to recognize what is important to you. Identifying your values will prepare you for setting personal and professional goals. Setting personal and professional goals helps you decide on the direction your practice must go. It guides you toward a mission statement.

45

# Setting Professional Goals

Circle your ideal response.

1. Participation in national organizations and associations:
   American Academy of Optometry, American Society of Cataract and Refractive Surgeons, American Public Health Association, National Academy of Opticianry, American Optometric Association, College of Vision Development, Optometric Extension Program, regional conferences, Better Vision Institute, American Optometric Foundation, American Academy of Ophthalmology, Optician's Association of America, Contact Lens Society of America, school alumni association, school faculty, school board of trustees, other _____

2. Participation in state organizations and associations committees:
   Board of trustees, education, health care delivery, public awareness, membership, legislative, PAC, Vision West Inc., other _____

3. State society activities:
   Society officer, education, membership, governmental affairs, PAC, bulletin, public awareness, other _____

4. Public service:
   Public speaking, writing articles, newspaper contact, political contact key person, school consultant, industrial consultant, expert witness, state board member, school board member, public health service, Flying Samaritans, VOSH, Vision USA, special Olympics, other _____

5. Professional services:
   Primary care, contact lenses, low vision, visual therapy, sports vision, geriatric vision, orthokeratology, pediatrics, traumatic brain injury, convalescent hospital care, hospital emergency

care, spectacles, finishing lab, full service lab, solutions, pre- and postop care, surgical procedures, other _____

6. In summary, my professional goals are

_____

_____

Review your personal and professional goals. Ask yourself, what impact does this have on my practice? What changes in my practice are necessary to facilitate reaching my goals? Use these needs to develop your ideal mission statement.

# Future Plans[19]

This exercise is designed to increase awareness of areas in which you have growth opportunities, assist you in identifying resources needed to carry out your plans, and encourage you to recognize those areas most consistent with your plans.

You should do this exercise throughout life; it can give you direction and motivate you to use your time constructively. The outline will help organize your dreams into concrete goals.

Some categories may not be relevant to you, and feel free to add more categories. Each goal is best expressed as measurable and specific. Include a target date for each. For each goal, write down where you are today, obstacles to achieving the goal, checkpoint dates, and specific actions to take to form new habits.

I. *Educational*
   a. Interest classes
   b. Postgraduate education

II. *Eyecare Practice*
   a. Self-employed or employed
   b. Location
   c. Type of practice
   d. Scope of practice

III. *Teaching*
   a. Public speaking
   b. City college
   c. University
   d. Optometry school

IV. *Research*
   a. Private practice
   b. Industry
   c. Optometry school

V. *Investments*
   a. Real estate
      1. Home
      2. Office
      3. Vacation home
   b. Practice
   c. Stocks and bonds
   d. Retirement
   e. Insurance
   f. Other

VI. *Home improvements/ construction*
   a. Interior decorating
   b. Landscaping

VII. *Personal*
   a. Cars
   b. Clothes
   c. Dining out
   d. Other

VIII. *Community activities*
   a. Church, temple
   b. Service clubs
   c. Other

IX. *Political office*
   a. Optometric
      1. Local
      2. State
      3. National
   b. Public
      1. Local
      2. State
      3. National
 X. *Travel*
   a. National
   b. International
XI. *Recreation*
   a. Sports
   b. Hobbies
   c. Club membership

XII. *Family*
   a. Marriage
   b. Children
   c. Children/spouse plans
XIII. *Retirement*
   a. When
   b. Expected income level
   c. Planned activities
   d. Location
      1. Local
      2. State

## Notes

1. Hamel G, Prahalad CK. Strategic intent. *Harvard Business Review.* 1989;67(3):63–76.
2. Ireland RD, Hitt M. Mission statements. *Business Horizons.* 1992;35(3):34–42.
3. Pearce J, David E. Corporate mission statements: The bottom line. *Academy of Management Executive.* 1987;1.
4. Abel D. *Defining the Business: The Starting Point of Strategic Planning.* Englewood Cliffs, NJ: Prentice-Hall; 1980.
5. Campbell A, Yeung S. *Do You Need a Mission Statement.* London: The Economist Publications; 1990.
6. Campbell A, Yeung S. Creating a sense of mission. *Long Range Planning.* 1991;24(4):10–20.
7. Wickman P. Developing a mission for an entrepreneurial venture. *Management Decision.* May–June 1997;35(5–6):373–381.
8. Levitt T. Marketing myopia. *Harvard Business Review.* July–August 1960:45–56.
9. Christopher M, Majaro S, McDonald M. *Strategy Search: A Guide to Marketing for Chief Executives and Directors.* Aldershot, England: Gower Press; 1987:8.
10. Baxter International. *Annual report.* 1993.
11. Bennis W. Becoming a nation of leaders. In: Toffler A, Toffler H, *Rethinking the Future.* London: Nicholas Brealey Publishing; 1997.
12. Stated during a "Pathways in Optometry" seminar delivered by Williams Consulting Group, Lincoln, NE, 1993.
13. Shaw-McMinn P. "Personal goal setting for ODs at all career stages. *Optometric Economics.* Spring 1996;6(2):20–21.
14. Act now—or die: Why you must plan beyond yourself to succeed today. *Success Magazine.* September 1989:50.
15. Evaluation and re-evaluation. *Ophthalmology Management.* March 5, 1989;5(3):24–25.
16. Yenawine G. Life Design Program seminars. Boston, 1986.
17. *Marketing News.* March 1, 1995:1.
18. Modified from Your business and financial plan, Module 1. *AOA Practice Enhancement Program,* course workbook. St. Louis, MO: American Optometric Assocation; 1986:9.
19. Shaw-McMinn P. Goal setting. *Optometric Economics.* Spring 1996;6(2):24.

# CHAPTER 3

# Analyzing Market Opportunities

If opportunity doesn't knock, build a door.

*—Anonymous*

One challenge with which many ECPs are consistently confronted is how to increase patient volume or local market share while attempting to decrease expenses by using fewer resources. Traditional advertising goals aim to appeal to the general population by creating awareness of the practice within the community and encouraging patients to return for regular care. The marketing needs of today's ECPs are different and more specific, requiring effective, measurable, and well-targeted tactics. **The consequences of adapting a myopic viewpoint (defining your services and mission too narrowly) could restrict your ability to reach potential target groups and stifle the growth of your business.**[1] Consider the difference between focusing on the "eyeglass" business as opposed to the "vision correction" business. The former limits what you are able to do by placing a limitation on the products offered. The latter opens up many more possibilities by simply expanding the product opportunities you offer consumers to correct their vision problems. Even further, "ocular wellness" adds the concept of prevention and goes beyond vision, greatly expanding what you are able to offer your patients.

Marketing analysis utilizes a variety of tools at the ECP's disposal, starting with information obtained from market research data. Next, the segmentation process identifies potential patients, while buyer behavior analysis alerts the ECP to products and services that potential patients desire. The actions taken by competitors in response to tactics the ECP initiates and opportunities suppliers offer play a significant part in the marketing strategy ultimately developed by the ECP.

## Market Research

Market research is the systematic acquisition of definitive answers to specific, relevant questions. The knowledge and understanding the ECP gains of his or her market is used in making projections and decisions. The primary function of market research is to provide answers to the following questions used by the ECP to develop a marketing plan:

1. What growth trends and changes are taking place that affect my practice?
2. Is there a pattern emerging that I can observe and might take advantage of to increase revenues or that might affect my practice in a negative manner, for which I should prepare?
3. How predictable are the changes that affect or control the way I operate my practice? And what is the likelihood that I can influence these events for future planning?
4. What patterns of growth, rate of change, and direction and sequence of events are influencing the ophthalmic industry?
5. What trends affect eyecare and the ophthalmic industry, now and in the future?
6. How predictable and useful are the trends that influence the way I create a business strategy and marketing plans?

The American Marketing Association defines the process of *market research* as the "link between consumer, customer, and public to the marketer through information used to identify and define marketing opportunities and problems; generate, refine and evaluate marketing actions; monitor marketing performance; and improve understanding of marketing as a process."[2] A study performed by the Academy for Health Services Marketing ranked the most common uses of the results of market research:[3]

1. Measure public image and patient awareness.
2. Gauge the potential for offering specific services.
3. Monitor key target segments.
4. Survey consumer preferences.
5. Assist strategic planning.
6. Monitor advertising effectiveness.

As the marketing strategist for your practice, you first scan the marketplace to identify what changes are occurring or may occur in the near future.[4] What potential opportunities exist of which you may take advantage? Are there any areas where you could be the first ECP to exclusively offer a specific brand of product or unique service, giving you a competitive advantage (first-mover opportunity)? Next, monitor marketplace changes in patient preferences and purchasing patterns.[5] If you can detect current or potential trends, these may present an advantage. Third, forecast and develop projections about the trends that might affect the choices of action for the practice.[5] Modifications or alternative actions should be planned accordingly. Finally, assess the relevance and impact of all these factors on the marketplace environment.[5]

The data on which you base decisions can be either primary or secondary. Primary data is new information obtained directly from your patients and their records. You can gather this information through observation, survey questionnaires, or in person through focus groups and telephone surveys. Figure 3–1 has sample questions an ECP can mail to patients when gathering primary data. Secondary data is information already compiled and obtained from outside sources. This typically is less expensive than obtaining new, primary data. The disadvantage is the variability in the degree of relevance this type of data may have to your particular practice.

## Analyzing the External Marketplace

Six components should be analyzed to understand the external marketplace in which the ECP operates: the demographic,

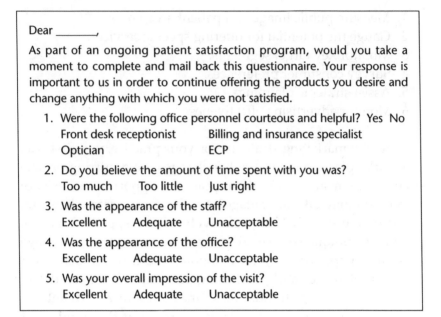

Dear _____,

As part of an ongoing patient satisfaction program, would you take a moment to complete and mail back this questionnaire. Your response is important to us in order to continue offering the products you desire and change anything with which you were not satisfied.

1. Were the following office personnel courteous and helpful? Yes No
   Front desk receptionist      Billing and insurance specialist
   Optician                     ECP

2. Do you believe the amount of time spent with you was?
   Too much      Too little      Just right

3. Was the appearance of the staff?
   Excellent      Adequate      Unacceptable

4. Was the appearance of the office?
   Excellent      Adequate      Unacceptable

5. Was your overall impression of the visit?
   Excellent      Adequate      Unacceptable

**Figure 3–1    Sample mail survey questionnaire**

economic, regulatory, sociocultural, technological, and global aspects.[6] These six components should be carefully examined to identify any trends or changes that will have a significant impact on the way you develop future business strategies? Typically, the demographic and sociocultural variables are the two with the greatest impact, because they change the most often and fastest, while the others are relatively stable and predictable. A thorough understanding of these components will allow you to anticipate threats to the practice's success and identify areas of opportunity.

### Demographic Influence

The demographic segment includes the size of the present and potential drawing population for your office, age breakdown of your patients, geographic distribution (usually categorized by zip code), ethnic mix, and income distribution of your patients.

Determine to which groups of patients to target your marketing, based on the population characteristics within the community.

As an example of how you might utilize this information in your practice, examine demographic data collected. The U.S. Census Bureau tells us that one third of the U.S. population was born between 1946 and 1964, and those over age 65 (34 million people) currently represent 13% of the total population. Projections show this segment will double by the year 2011, with the first baby boomers becoming eligible for Medicare. According to *American Demographics* magazine, the segment over age 45 spends 17% more than the average American household, while the primary advertising target, those between the age of 25 and 34, actually spend 13% less.[7]

In 1957, the annual birth rate was at the peak of the baby boom segment with 4.3 million births that year. The lowest rate was in 1976 with 3.2 million births but has steadily increased since then. The annual birth rate has been stable at about 4 million births per year since 1990. Using this information offers the prospect of a new generation of strong pediatric demand, given the greater number of births over the past decade. The segment of the population over age 85 represents 3.5% of the total population; this is up 274% since 1960 and will double by the year 2020. This group requires eyecare services four times more than other segments of the population. What does this mean to you? And how do you use this information in your strategic planning?

One assumption is that the number of future patients eligible for Medicare will increase, given the present trend. Due to the decrease in nursing home residents, this might be a specialty area where the competition becomes increasingly more difficult over time. Another assumption is that the relatively stable and greater number of new births during the past decade makes the demand for a pediatric specialty more favorable. Both are examples of the type of data that you could collect and how it might affect your practice planning. Birth rate and demographic information can be obtained from various commercial clearinghouses, your local library (ask for Burwell's *Directory of Information Brokers*), and several government sources.[8]

## Effect of the Economy

The second component involves economics, including the levels and trends of key indicators, such as interest rates, that affect your ability to borrow funds to expand your practice. Also, the consumer price index (CPI), which reflects the inflation rate, exerts an influence on your patients' ability and willingness to seek your services. With higher inflation, patients may be more apt to postpone visits to the ECP. A recent study by the Employee Benefit Research Institute concluded that 22 percent of adults who do not have health insurance have annual incomes over $50,000.[9] This group offers the ECP the opportunity to develop unique individual eyecare plans for this level of uninsured families. Information regarding economic forecasting is quite technical in nature and beyond the scope of this book, but it can be obtained on the Internet.[10]

## Regulatory Agencies

The third part of the external analysis is the impact that political, legal, and regulatory change will have on the way you practice. This normally affects ECPs as an entire profession or on a large, regional basis. Are there pending regulations with potential to influence the profitability of your practice? The Institute for Health Care Strategies has suggested that HMO-managed care will level off at a national penetration of 37%; however, continued growth will occur in both Medicare and Medicaid markets.[11] This is good for ECPs because of the input that professional eyecare groups can exert on the governing bodies that administer Medicare and Medicaid, as opposed to private HMO business decision makers. In addition, government-supported fees typically are higher than HMO-managed care fees. Are there legal barriers or obstacles, such as specific regulations, that could either prevent or enhance your ability to pursue a specific strategy? Active involvement in local societies is the best way to keep abreast of the changes affecting the eyecare profession.

## Trends in Society

Sociocultural factors, the fourth area, includes changing patient attitudes that affect your practice, such as future changes in employer-sponsored health coverage from a defined benefit to a defined contribution. How do changing social attitudes and cultural values held by patients affect the ECP's marketing strategy? What changes should be anticipated and accounted for to remain competitive? Adding to the demographic component, will attitudes of the growing segment of older Americans produce an "age wave" cultural shift away from youth toward the needs and concerns of the middle-aged and senior set?

An example of a sociocultural trend advantageous to ECPs was reported in a recent study, which showed patient visits to alternative and complementary providers increased 47% from 1990 to 1997.[12] To develop this "extension" as a meaningful source of revenue, the promotions you use must first educate patients as to the benefits they would receive through in-office seminars, video presentations, or bundled with other promotional materials. You can emphasize the convenience of "all-in-one shopping" and the importance of monitoring progress through the eye health record the office has generated. Additional support can be offered by giving patients copies of studies that attest to "the importance of proper nutrition and how supplements that detoxify the body can help slow cataract progression and macular degeneration."[13] However, recommending and selling ocular vitamin therapy regimens places the ECP in a highly aggressive environment, "competing against every corner grocery store, vitamin store, and others that exist in your community."[12]

### Impact of Technology

The fifth segment of the external analysis is technology, which accounts for the different ways new knowledge or processes can be applied to change or affect the ECP's practice operations and systems. Could any newly developed technology or new communication method threaten or enhance patient loyalty? Could the discovery of a genetic link as the cause of refractive error affect the way ECPs practice in the future? How will changes in marketing technology affect the way patients find you? The increased amount of refractive surgery marketing will have a definite short-term impact on patient decision making. What can you do to prevent any unwanted effect on practice revenue or disruption patient flow from the rapid growth and consolidation in this area?

### Global Influence

The final contributing element to the ECP's external market analysis presently has the least impact. Global forces have not exerted much influence on the status of ECPs in the United States to date. Both international academic and ophthalmic industry alliances have been established during the past decade, but no trends from outside this country have had any significant domestic impact. However, with trade and research alliances being formed between North American, European, and Asian nations, the introduction of new competing foreign technologies into this country may accelerate.

## Future Planning

At best, long-range planning is an educated guess. Any concrete strategies for implementation beyond 3 years should have definite contingencies and a best-worst case scenario analysis. Market research seeks definitive answers to specific questions for a more in-depth understanding of unfamiliar marketplace conditions. Your decisions are based on the information and data obtained; therefore, the more relevant and specific the information is to your unique situation, the more valuable. This information often can be elusive and costly to obtain but certainly necessary for proper decision making. Northwestern University Business School professor and marketing consultant Philip Kotler offers suggestions on characteristics of health care consumers and their wants for the new millennium, as described in Table 3–1.[14] These are the result of extensive market research and some of the suggestions listed should be considered driving forces for changing the present methods you use to operate your practice.

Assessing your local drawing area's potential, opportunities for and sources of the most likely patient groups to seek your

**Table 3–1    Characteristics of Health Care Consumers**

1. Seniors over age 50 will become primary purchasers of products and services.
2. People want entertainment when working, shopping, or consuming.
3. Marketing tactics will need to stress personalized service and high-quality products.
4. Basic, not lavish, least-cost products and services will gain popularity with a shrinking middle class.
5. Consumers will frequent providers offering more convenience.
6. Patient relations and segmentation will be made easier with the use of computer analysis.

Modified from Kotler P. *Kotler on Marketing*. New York: Free Press; 1999.

services can be a valuable exercise in predicting profitability. Appendix 3–1 offers various ways to assess your particular community's potential, while Appendix 3–2 lists the activities and organizations that offer ECPs opportunities to promote their practice. An in-office project for assignment to a staff member (shown in Appendix 3–3) will help you identify the patients most likely to refer other patients to you. Finally, Appendix 3–4 lists health care agencies that might refer potential patients to your practice. The external marketplace affects all ECPs in your drawing area equally; however, those competitors that have a better understanding of current trends can anticipate and adapt faster when change is required.

## SWOT Analysis

A useful tool for understanding your practice, competition, and external market environment is a SWOT analysis. This reveals the strengths and weaknesses (SW) of your office (internal) as well as the opportunities and threats (OT) of the current social, legal, economic, and regulatory climate (external) that could limit what you are able to achieve. A list of questions to analyze your current situation is found in Table 3–2.[15]

One reference that compiles sources to answer SWOT developed questions can be found in "A Guide to Finding and Evaluating Best Practices Health Care Information."[16] According to a 1998 American Academy of Ophthalmology projection, the demand for eyecare services is predicted to adequately increase in the near future.[17] Table 3–3 projects a future increase in demand for the higher-reimbursing Evaluation and Management (E&M) coding methods, which are relatively new for ECPs, but allows revenue to be maximized through proper documentation and use of the more medically specific 99000 E&M codes.

Tremendous opportunity exists in the area of low vision, using recently released statistics from three independent sources. The low-vision market will grow at a cumulative annual growth rate of 10% or greater to the year 2007,[18] while a recent AOA survey showed a nearly 45% drop in the number of providers performing low-vision services since 1987.[19] Research from the respected low-vision resource the Lighthouse projects the number of baby boomers with moderate and severe vision loss will increase by 1.4 million by the end of this decade.[20] Obviously, this is one area that exhibits great opportunity for many new providers to enter.

## Competitor Analysis

Tactics to gain information about your competitors have been considered ethically arguable by some, but this is not always the case. Fortunately, we are in an industry in which professional espionage has not yet become necessary; demand remains strong even though the supply of ECPs is disproportionate to the population in some regions. However, valuable information includes knowing the characteristics of the major competitors in your area and their present and potential performance. What new strategies might future competitors use? Posing questions to a current patient who was formerly examined by one of your competitors is one tactic you can use to gain information. An even more aggressive approach is to send someone into a competitor's office

## Table 3–2    SWOT Analysis

*Internal Conditions*

Strengths
    Does the office run efficiently?
    Is the staff skilled and knowledgeable?
    Do I have sufficient funds budgeted to accomplish my goals?
    Is the office reputation superior?
    Is my mission statement and purpose well stated and understood?

Weaknesses
    Is my strategy and direction unclear?
    Is the equipment old or obsolete?
    Do I have staff problems and constant turnover?
    Is the office image weak?
    Do I exhibit below average marketing skills?
    Do we offer an inadequate number and assortment of services and products?

*External Conditions*

Opportunities
    Are there possible new target markets?
    Can we diversify by offering new services or products?
    Can we expand coverage either geographically or in hours of service?

Threats
    Are there new competitive entrants?
    Are there substitute services?
    Are consumers' tastes changing?
    Will regulatory agencies impose restrictions?
    How will closed panels affect me?

*Additional Questions*

What trends effect the way I earn revenue and make profits and why?

Is my revenue linked to the quality of the product and services I deliver, my marketing program effectiveness, the efficient utilization of resources in my practice, or some combination of all three factors?

What is really important for an ECP to do well to be successful?

What benchmarks should I be watching (using data to identify the methods high-performance practices use)?

What makes better practices profitable?

Modified with permission from Stone B. Strategic marketing and communications audits. *Journal of Health Care Marketing.* Winter 1995;15(4):54–56.

**Table 3–3    Future Demand for Eye Care**

| CPT Code | Service Description | Projected Increase |
|---|---|---|
| 92000 (eye exam codes) | Eye exams and lens fittings | +4–10% |
| 99000 (medical codes) | Office visits and consultations | +14–16% |

posing as a patient to gain firsthand knowledge, although this may be considered a bit extreme, if not unethical.

The easiest way to obtain competitor intelligence is to diligently monitor the media in your area and compile profiles on your competition's marketing. Select two or three service providers considered to be your major competitors and complete Appendix 3–5 to gain a better understanding of the status of other providers. This is one of the best tools you have for evaluating and planning your practice enhancement strategies, because it allows you to offer services different from your competitors and claim unoccupied market positions, a primary component of practice image development. Several sources listed in Table 3–4 offer this type of information.

The ECP who performs diligent, concerted market research, analyzing both internal and external market influences, will be in a better position to systematically plan and execute a cost-efficient marketing and business strategy. Once that strategy is initiated, the ECP may begin to identify target groups of patients

**Table 3–4    Sources for Information About Competitors**

1. Your own knowledge, experience, and impressions.
2. Feedback from patients who have switched to your practice.
3. Professional contacts with other service providers.
4. Sales representatives.
5. Fellow ECPs themselves.
6. Community members.
7. Staff members who formerly worked for other ECPs.
8. Staff members.

most likely to utilize the services his or her practice offers; this is addressed in Chapter 4.

> When you come to a fork in the road, take it.
>
> —*Yogi Berra*

## Action Plan for ECPs

1. Identify resources and people that offer useful, analytic current information about your local community.
2. Complete the Community Analysis exercise to determine specific information and knowledge about your local community (Appendix 3–1).
3. Complete the Community Activities Checklist to assist you in ranking potential opportunities to explore as sources of new revenue (Appendix 3–2).
4. Complete the Patient Referral Sources exercise to determine where your patients are coming from (Appendix 3–3).
5. Examine Referral Agency Sources list to select community organizations and agencies with which you may want to form alliances (Appendix 3–4).
6. Complete the Competitor Service Provider Data Form to classify the level of competition in your area (Appendix 3–5).
7. Identify those competitors that pursue marketing the most aggressively. What are they doing that you should be doing but presently are not?
8. Decide on a strategy to use to compete with your competitors.

# Community Analysis

The purpose of this community assessment is to identify and organize certain facts about your practice community. From it you can get a realistic picture of the potential of your community for patients. The following sources may be used to get the information: local library; Chamber of Commerce; city, town, and county planners (offices or committees); superintendent of schools; social agencies; local telephone books.

Estimated population _____

Percentage of age group mix:

    Infants (birth–4 years) _____

    School-aged children _____

    Young adults _____

    Adults (26–40) _____

    Middle aged (41–60) _____

    Older adults (61+) _____

Approximate annual income _____

Percent of ethnic/racial mix _____

Number of persons employed _____

Number unemployed _____

Major employers _____

Types of work

    Retail sales _____

    Professional/technical _____

    Computer _____

    Heavy manufacturing _____

    Light industrial _____

    Clerical _____

    Government _____

    Homemaking _____

    Education _____

Number of families _____

Number of households _____

Cost of housing (range) _____

    Home ownership _____

    Rental _____

Percent of homeowners _____

Type of transportation available

_____

Number of office complexes _____

Number of businesses _____

Number of industries _____

Types of industries _____

Number of senior citizen housing _____

Number of nursing homes _____

Hospitals, medical centers, clinics _____

Names of community leaders

_____

_____

_____

_____

_____

_____

| | | |
|---|---|---|
| Self-employed | _____ | Names of social leaders |
| Executive/management | _____ | _____ |
| Other (specify) | _____ | _____ |
| Estimated school enrollment | | _____ |
| Preschool | _____ | _____ |
| Elementary (K–6) | _____ | _____ |
| Middle school (7–9) | _____ | _____ |
| High school (10–12) | _____ | |
| Trade school | _____ | Projected changes |
| College and university | _____ | Residential _____ |
| | | Business _____ |
| | | Industrial _____ |
| | | School _____ |

# Community Activities Checklist

This checklist lists common community organizations. Identify those to which you belong by checking the Member column. Check the Active column if you actively participate in the organization's activities or are a committee member or officer. Check whether the organization is primarily in your practice community or your home community. List any others you can think of.

| Organization | Member | Active | Near Practice | Near Home |
|---|---|---|---|---|
| Church | | | | |
| Temple | | | | |
| Religious organization | | | | |
| Chamber of Commerce | | | | |
| Rotary | | | | |
| Kiwanis | | | | |
| Elks | | | | |
| Odd Fellows | | | | |
| Shriners, Masons | | | | |
| School related: PTA, boosters, athletic, etc. | | | | |
| Fraternity or sorority | | | | |
| College alumni | | | | |
| YMCA or YWCA | | | | |
| Women's club | | | | |
| Newcomer's club | | | | |
| Country club | | | | |
| Athletic club | | | | |
| Business or professional club | | | | |

| Organization | Member | Active | Near Practice | Near Home |
|---|---|---|---|---|
| Eyecare society | | | | |
| Health or fitness club | | | | |
| VFW, American Legion | | | | |
| Historical society | | | | |
| Lions Club | | | | |
| Optimists | | | | |
| Altrusa | | | | |
| Scout groups | | | | |
| Toastmasters | | | | |
| League of Women Voters | | | | |
| Elected or appointed board (park, library, school) | | | | |
| Political office | | | | |
| Other (specify) | | | | |

# APPENDIX 3–3

# Patient Referral Sources

Ask a staff member to pull the patient record cards for 100 current patients whom you have seen in the last 6 months. Tally the information according to the following list. This will give you an idea of who refers patients to you. Many computer programs can assist you in collecting this information.

| Source of Referral | Number of Patients |
|---|---|
| Other family member(s) who are already patients | |
| Friend or business associate who is your patient | |
| Other professional: | |
|    Teacher | |
|    Psychologist | |
|    School nurse | |
|    Physician | |
|    Other optometrist | |
|    Optician | |
|    Ophthalmologist | |
|    Other (specify) | |
| Contact through organizations to which I belong | |
| Contact through organizations to which family members or friends belong | |
| Managed-care organization | |
|    HMO | |
|    PPO | |
|    MSO | |

| *Source of Referral* | *Number of Patients* |
|---|---|
| Walk-ins | |
| Articles written about me | |
| Yellow page telephone listing | |
| Speeches I have given | |
| Current staff | |
| Social contacts | |
| Website | |
| Other (specify) | |

# APPENDIX 3–4

# Referral Agency Sources

The following list specifies health care agencies that might refer patients to you. Check the ones that exist in your community and those that currently refer patients to you. Add to the list any others in your community.

| Agency | Exists | Refers |
|---|---|---|
| Hospital | | |
| Physician group | | |
| School nurse | | |
| Nursing home | | |
| HMO | | |
| Older adult center | | |
| YMCA or YWCA | | |
| Agency for the multiply handicapped | | |
| Commission for the blind | | |
| Department of children and family services | | |
| Children's group home | | |
| Other county agency | | |
| Other city agency | | |
| Other state agency | | |
| Urgent care center | | |
| Senior citizen center | | |
| Other (specify) | | |

# Competitor Service Provider Data Form

Use this form to collect details about other providers in your area. Make comparisons to what you presently are or are not doing in your practice.

Name of provider: _____ Date: _____

Address and telephone:_____
_____

Major patient groups: _____
_____

Directly competing services:_____
_____

New services being developed: _____

Public image and positioning with patients: _____
_____

Community or public service group affiliations:_____
_____

Major strengths: _____
_____

Major weaknesses: _____
_____

How does this provider inform the potential patients about his or her services? (Promotion or public education activities) _____

_____

_____

What's different about your practice and this provider's practice? How can you best exploit the difference? _____

_____

## Notes

1. Levitt T. Marketing myopia. *Harvard Business Review.* July–
   August 1960:45–56.
2. Bennett P. *Dictionary of Marketing Terms.* Chicago: American
   Marketing Association; 1988.
3. Marlowe D. *Building a Foundation for Effective Healthcare Market Research.* Chicago: Academy for Health Services Marketing; 1990.
4. Elenkov D. Strategic uncertainty and environmental scan-
   ning. *Strategic Management Journal.* 1997;18:287–313.
5. Fahey L, Narayanan V. *Macroenvironmental Analysis for
   Strategic Management.* St. Paul, MN: West Publishing; 1986:
   39–42
6. Hitt M, Ireland R, Hoskisson R. *Strategic Management.* 4th ed.
   Cincinatti: South-Western College Publishing; 2001:56–66.
7. DeLong S. Retail beat. *Eyecare Business.* January 1998:12.
8. Sources include Find/SVP at 212-645-4500 and the American Marketing Association at 312-648-0536, which offers the
   *International Directory of Marketing Research Companies and
   Services.*
9. Eye openers. *InSight Washington.* May 5, 2000:4.
10. Twice a year, refer to www. firstunion.com/econews(basic
    statistics) and www.cbo.gov/byclass.cfm, the website of the
    Congressional Budget Office that projects an economic out-
    look.
11. Moore P. Accept change, control what you can. *MGMA Up-
    date.* January 15, 2000;39(2):1–3.
12. Dunevitz B. Alternative medicine a market opportunity.
    *Medical Group Management Update.* February 1, 2000:6.
13. Fundinglands B. Complementary commentary. *EyeWorld.*
    July 1999:15.
14. Kotler P. *Kotler on Marketing.* New York: Free Press; 1999.
15. Suggested from Stone B. Strategic marketing and communi-
    cations audits. *Journal of Health Care Marketing.* Winter 1995;
    15(4):54–56.
16. Published by the Joint Commission Journal on Quality Im-
    provement, phone 218-723-9477.

17. Beiting J. The Balanced Budget Act: How it impacts our bottom line. *Eyeworld*. October 1997:22.
18. Croft W. Getting the word out. *Eyecare Business*. December 1998:26.
19. Optometry then . . . and now. *AOA News*. 38(12):6.
20. Figures extrapolated from Croft W. Spreading the word. *Eyecare Business*. February 2000;15(2):50–52.

# CHAPTER 4

# Identifying and Targeting Patients

> I was seldom able to see an opportunity until it ceased to
> be one.                                                    —*Mark Twain*

## Identifying Segments

A market consists of a set of potential purchasers sharing a common need.[1] A segment for the ECP's office is a subset of a market or group of potential patients sharing common characteristics and common needs who are similar in the way they purchase, value, perceive, and use specific products or services. The segmentation process starts by dividing the market into groups with similar characteristics, then selecting the most appropriate to serve. There are at least eight different consumer types, each accounting for 8–17% of the population, from which 65 psychological dimensions can be simplified to 15 attributes that together are used to predict consumer behavior.[2] The six most often-used variables to identify segments for health care settings are these:

1. Personal characteristics (demographic).
2. Buyer behavior (psychographic).
3. Geographic location.
4. Lifestyle needs and use.
5. Benefits desired (attitude toward specific products).
6. Entitlements (insurance coverage).

Identifying the patients to target through the segmentation process can be facilitated by dividing the most likely parameters the ECP may use into defined groups. As an example, the behavioral aspect of the patient market can be divided into several components, including patients' needs, benefits gained through use, frequency of use, brand appeal, and information required. The demographic variable typically is easier for the ECP to identify. These include income level, age, gender, education level, ethnic group, social class, family size, and life-cycle phase.[3]

Appendix 4–1 will help you recognize the types of patients you presently target. You may be surprised to discover what types of patients you actually do attract, possibly unknowingly. Appendix 4–2 helps identify groups of patients you feel you would like to target.[4] Compare the differences in your results between the two exercises.

Using patient *needs* as the segmenting variable, you can break down the category into patients with a functional need (1-day contact lenses to satisfy a specific need such as a social event or backups to wear in event of loss), psychological need concerning personal appearance (a designer-style frame to gain an executive look), or a physiological need (ametropia causing blurred vision). Another variable used to identify or segment specific patient groups is the *benefits desired* by patients when they use a product or service. Is the benefit functional (to satisfy a visual impairment), situational (specific for advantages gained during certain events such as seeing a concert), or general (using spectacles to improve the overall quality of life)? Benefits that patients seek can be divided into four groups[5]:

1. *Quality.* The patient wants the best eyecare and is not concerned with cost.
2. *Service.* The patient wants a caring, personal attitude from the ECP.
3. *Value.* The patient wants the ECP that has a "reasonable" image and "reasonable" costs.
4. *Economy.* The patient wants the least expensive eyecare and is not as concerned with quality or quantity.

*Usage rate* is another variable by which you can identify a more finite group of patients to target for marketing. Patients may use certain products often (1-day disposable contacts) or constantly (extended wear contacts), infrequently or occasionally (colored contacts for socials) or rarely (disposable contact lenses for vacations only). *Brand appeal* is a factor because certain patients insist on using only a specific brand (either from positive prior experience, the recommendation of someone they trust, or aggressive marketing), others have a preference for one brand over another (these patients probably seek additional information), still others recognize but do not favor any particular brand (these patients will allow the ECP to choose), and finally some patients object to or refuse to use a specific brand (possibly from prior negative experience). The *information* patients require to make a purchasing decision can be classified as extensive (supported by expert documentation or medical studies), moderate (having heard or read about the product several times), or light (a one-time recommendation).

On successful completion of the preparation phase, including a careful analysis of both your situation and the marketplace, the next step is to formulate a plan by identifying groups of patients to target in your marketing tactics. To properly identify these various patient groups, the ECP must have adequate data obtained from market research. Table 4–1 shows one method of dividing the population for marketing purposes.[6] Once sufficiently familiar with consumer characteristics, you can begin to separate the market into similar groups, according to your marketing programs. These questions should be answered before you start the segmentation process:

1. How frequently do patients use your services?
2. What media reach these potential patients?
3. How important is brand loyalty to patients?
4. Why do patients purchase your services?

## Segmentation Process

Demographics, using either income level or social class as a variable, can be separated according to the ECP's choice into low, middle, upper, low middle, upper middle, low upper, and so forth. Age can be broken down by quantifiable numeric groups using

Table 4–1    Example of Sociocultural Segmentation
for Marketing Purposes

| Segment | Percent | Description |
|---|---|---|
| Traditional populist | 15 | Working class, men, less than 45 years old |
| Steward | 15 | Retired, affluent, college educated |
| Dowagers | 7 | Elderly women, few attended college |
| Liberal activist | 20 | Young, college educated, single |
| Conservative activist | 15 | Two thirds are men, college educated with children and high incomes |
| Ethnic conservative | 16 | Two thirds are women, older, few attended college, low incomes |
| Agnostics | 12 | Older Baby Boomers, high incomes |

Adapted from Selbert. *U.S. News & World Report.* 1995:3.

scores of years (0–20, 20–40, 40–60, or over 60) or by qualitative groupings (youths, young adults, adults, seniors). Family cycles include single, married, married with or without children, and empty nest or divorced. Current demographic and census studies reveal that, due to larger numbers of immigrants entering this country, ethnic groups are the fastest-growing segments of the U.S. economy. Identifying these groups and marketing specifically to their needs can offer advantages to ECPs. As an example, certain Asian groups have higher incidences of myopia, while certain South Americans exhibit hyperopia and become presbyopic at a younger age. **Marketing messages of an informative nature related specifically to symptoms these groups may experience would be appropriate and prove beneficial, especially using a media that targets the specific groups you want to reach.**

Using demographic parameters is a simple, yet effective method to narrow your selection of marketing tactics to reach patients. Choosing two parameters—for example, gender and income—results in six distinct groups: females and males with either low, medium, or high incomes. Next, choose one of these six groups as your target group. Decide the best way to utilize the four Ps (price, promotion, product, and place) discussed in Chapter 6) to develop your marketing mix's appeal to this select group. Replace one of the demographic parameters with a psychographic variable, such as perceived impact of contact lenses on a patient's social life. This could yield many groups: patients concerned with functional benefits, youthful appearance, and so on. How does this affect your previous choice of the marketing mix? Would you have to redesign your marketing message or channels to appeal to this new target group? Finally, replace one of the parameters with a lifestyle usage variable, such as part-time wearers of contact lenses, sports enthusiasts, or occupational requirements. How does this new segment influence the design of your marketing strategy?

It is possible that one particular marketing mix may be favorable to reach several different segments. In that case, if there are certain tactics that might reach more than one segment you might find it more cost effective to use that particular marketing medium or channel. Each different segmentation parameter chosen has a unique influence in the way it affects the final design of the marketing mix you use to promote services to patients.[3]

For segmentation to be effective, members of each segment must be internally homogeneous and the distinctions between segments clear, well defined, and externally heterogeneous. An ideal segmentation strategy should maximize the difference between each of the segments created but minimize the difference within each segment in terms of chosen characteristics.[7] Members of each segment must be identifiable and reachable by methods within your means or your marketing efforts will be in vain. However, merely dividing your market into distinctly identifiable groups does not guarantee success. Segmentation is not sufficiently predictive by itself but requires a tracking mechanism to ensure the identified targets are contacted (see Chapter 6). Targeting requires you to choose viable groups to reach from the segments you identified. After evaluating the attractiveness and cost effectiveness of contacting the identified targets, you may decide to rule out certain groups because of the excessive cost to reach them in relation to the anticipated return on your marketing investment.

## Cluster Analysis

Another technique used to identify segments the ECP may target is called *cluster analysis*. Information from patients is compiled to form groups that have common characteristics. These similarities include past buying behavior, attitude toward certain products, specific needs, and benefits gained by using certain products. A cluster analysis of the contact lens market might reveal that some patients buy contacts because they believe they see better with contacts than glasses (pragmatic segment). Others may feel contacts offer a youthful appearance (lifestyle segment), while another group needs the safety benefits gained by contacts (benefits segment). After studying isolated segments, new and more effective methods of marketing to these select patient groups may become evident.[8]

Three segments for marketers that are prevalent and reachable are Baby Boomers (patients born from 1946 to 1964), Generation X patients (born from 1965 to 1978), and Generation Y patients (born from 1979 to 1994). Because vastly different social and economic factors influenced the development of these three segments, they do not share the same frame of reference regarding customer service and require different tactics for creating an appealing marketing message. Baby Boomers typically are not as comfortable using the Internet for purchasing products, unlike Generation Xers. Also, Baby Boomers relate to nostalgia in advertisements, while Generation Xers are suspicious of slick images; however, both groups dislike any noticeable amount of stress during their purchase decision making.[9] Generation Y are the children of Baby Boomers and, numbering 60 million, are almost four times as large as the 17 million of Generation X. Generation Y is more racially diverse, one third being nonwhite, one fourth living in single-parent homes, and three fourths having working mothers.[10] At present, the most successful marketing reaches the segment where members of this group gather, either on the Internet, at sport events, or on cable TV. This group is prime for the ECP to reach through websites or at scholastic sports outings.

## Positioning Your Products and Services in the Community

Once you have completed the targeting process, you are ready to position the products and services you offer. Requirements for successful product and service positioning are (1) be believable, (2) fit your overall practice mission, (3) be accepted and actively promoted by your staff, and (4) be long lasting, not a transient fad.

The position you want your services and products to occupy in the community comes from the positioning statement. This states how you wish your practice's products and services to be perceived by patients within the niches in which you want to compete.[11] Where do you want your practice to fit into your local marketplace? Given whatever information and knowledge is available, patients will rank all the ECPs they consider, based on their "perception of value which is a composite of quality, price, availability and service."[12] It is recommended that you adhere to the "Law of Focus" by Trout and Reis, that differentiation is vital when developing a positioning statement and try to narrow rather than broaden the qualities you will emphasize.[13] The short statement in Appendix 4–3 has been used for years by marketing professionals to develop a position statement.[14] You can start the process of creating your own brand identity by completing it.

## Focus Group Surveys and Sampling

The goal of a patient focus group survey is to ascertain how those you believe are important to your business feel about something, while the goal of sampling is to determine who to ask to make assumptions about what everyone thinks.[15] The groups you select should reflect your target population as a whole in order to make more informed decisions. Results using both probability and nonprobability samples always are interpreted with confidence levels or error ranges to allow for uncertainties in the process and with data collection.

The first category, probability sampling, is characterized by random selection with everyone in the group having an equal chance. The advantage is that results usually are unbiased and easily obtained. The disadvantage comes from the possibility of excluding relevant subgroups.[16] If desired, the population can be further divided into subgroups, then a random subgroup sample selection is made. This is used when an ECP wants to find out more about two groups, such as high-volume users of the office, one group between the ages of 25 and 45 and the second group over 65. A random sample is likely not to adequately represent the over 65 because it could be a significantly smaller group. Another type of probability sample, called *systematic sampling*, consists of assembling random groups and then pulling names using a predetermined ratio of population to the desired sample.[16] For example, if you want to send surveys to 200 people on a 1,000 person sample, select every fifth person (an example of Nth number sampling) and mail that person a survey. Finally, cluster sampling can be used: select random streets in a specific zip code and send everyone listed a survey.

Nonprobability sampling, based on survey needs, sometimes is reserved for difficult-to-find or specific groups.[16] This type often is used at the onset or start-up phase of a marketing program. Nonprobability sampling is chosen for convenience because of its ease of assembling, but it has the downside of possibly not generalizing to the desired target population. Under this category is snowball sampling: selecting additional group members identified by previously chosen members with the desired characteristic. An example would be a focus group of all presbyopic golfers for whom you wish to survey the potential benefit of a specific ophthalmic product. You believe your sample size is insufficient. Using this method, the ECP would ask members of a group to suggest names of additional presbyopic golfers they know to enlarge the sample size.

Errors always can hinder your interpretation and the ultimate application of the results. These may come from several sources. Duplication of names increases the likelihood of selecting or excluding people. An inaccurate description of a subgroup or an extraordinarily large percentage of nonrespondents skews the results. The choice of the actual sample size can be determined by imitating what others have used, choosing whatever is the most convenient and affordable for your purpose, or considering the level of accuracy and confidence level you require.[16]

**Patients**

|  | Current | Potential |
|---|---|---|
| **Current** | Offer | Develop |
| **Potential** | Acquire Ability | Diversify |

Products/Service

**Figure 4–1** **Strategic marketing choices, the options an ECP has with the products or services that a practice offers as a function of present or new patients.**

Once you have obtained a picture of what current and potential patients in your area want from your practice, you can decide which services to emphasize and which to eliminate. Figure 4–1 shows the options for the strategic business decision of offering products and services to current or potential patients. After you have identified patient target groups, the next step is to concentrate on developing and retaining lifetime patients, using a relationship marketing strategy—the topic of the next chapter.

## Action Plan for ECPs

1. Complete the Present Patient Profile in Appendix 4–1 to identify and develop patient groups that use your services with the most frequency.
2. Complete the Ideal Patient Profile to select groups of patients you want to use your services (Appendix 4–2).
3. Compare the results of these profiles to the local community population demographics that you determined in Chapter 3.
4. Identify target populations to use in your marketing plan.
5. Develop a position statement for various target groups (Appendix 4–3).

# Present Patient Profile

You can gain valuable insight about how to market your practice more effectively by reviewing your patients' charts. In fact, your files are a veritable gold mine, just waiting to tell you who your patients are, where they come from, and which of your services are most needed or underutilized. You also can use this information to spot trends in your patient population. For example, you may find that you see a high percentage of elderly patients but relatively few teenagers. Or you may discover that you're not fitting as many contact lenses as you might be.

Unearthing this valuable information is not difficult. Practice management consultants call the process *developing a patient profile*. While the terminology may sound forbidding, the procedure is not. All you have to do is complete the patient profile that follows for a random sample of 100 of your patients. To get a random sample, use your alphabetical listing of patients. Take the first 20 active patients under five letters of the alphabet such as A, C, D, M, and W, until you have a sample of 100. You may need to add another letter from which to take patient names for the sample.

To collect the required information, ask your staff to

1. Write the name of each patient on the patient profile.
2. Check the appropriate descriptions of each patient shown on the patient profile.
3. Tally the data in the total row.

**Patient Profile**

| Patient's Name | Sex | Age Cohort | | | | | Occupation | | | | | | | Service Rendered (by code number) | | | | | Location (by quadrant or zip code) | | | |
|---|---|---|---|---|---|---|---|---|---|---|---|---|---|---|---|---|---|---|---|---|---|---|
| | | 1–17 | 18–24 | 25–54 | 55–65 | 65+ | Blue Collar | White Collar | Homemaker | Professional | Retired | Student | Unemployed | 1 | 2 | 3 | 4 | 5 | 1 | 2 | 3 | 4 |
| | | | | | | | | | | | | | | | | | | | | | | |
| | | | | | | | | | | | | | | | | | | | | | | |
| | | | | | | | | | | | | | | | | | | | | | | |
| | | | | | | | | | | | | | | | | | | | | | | |
| | | | | | | | | | | | | | | | | | | | | | | |
| | | | | | | | | | | | | | | | | | | | | | | |
| | | | | | | | | | | | | | | | | | | | | | | |
| | | | | | | | | | | | | | | | | | | | | | | |
| | | | | | | | | | | | | | | | | | | | | | | |
| | | | | | | | | | | | | | | | | | | | | | | |
| Total | | | | | | | | | | | | | | | | | | | | | | |

Sample service codes: 1 = Diagnostic examination; 2 = Contact lenses; 3 = Low vision; 4 = Vision therapy; 5 = Glasses dispensed.

85

# Ideal Patient Profile

Complete the following checklist quickly, without analyzing your responses, so that you check your first, most instinctive, emotional reaction. Remember you're making this identification based on your feelings. Place a check in the Like column for those patients whom you like to see; in the Dislike column, for those whom you prefer not to see frequently; and in the Doesn't Matter column if you have no feelings one way or the other. If you would like more patients of a particular type put a plus in Wants column or a minus for those you would prefer to see fewer of.

| Patient | Like | Dislike | Doesn't Matter | Wants More, Fewer |
|---|---|---|---|---|
| Infants | | | | |
| Preschoolers | | | | |
| School-aged children | | | | |
| Adolescents | | | | |
| Young adults (20–39) | | | | |
| Middle aged (40–59) | | | | |
| Older adults (60+) | | | | |
| Married individuals | | | | |
| Single individuals | | | | |
| Single parents | | | | |
| Families | | | | |
| Business, career persons | | | | |
| Handicapped individuals | | | | |
| Nursing home residents | | | | |

| Patient | Like | Dislike | Doesn't Matter | Wants More, Fewer |
|---------|------|---------|----------------|-------------------|
| Non-English Speaking | | | | |
| Other (specify) | | | | |

Modified from Your marketing plan. AOA Practice Enhancement Program II, precourse workbook. St. Louis, MO: American Optometric Association; 1986.

# Developing a Position Statement[14]

You may want to reach multiple target groups; however, it is unlikely that the same positioning statement would appeal to several groups. In this case, you may wish to use more than one statement. You should only choose one brand category to market to each group, since multiple identity claims may result in your targets becoming confused. Your practice can be primary care, specialty care, high tech, family oriented, lowest price, and so forth. Make sure the unique service you lay claim to is not already being marketed by your competitors. There usually is only one leader, typically the one who markets first. The justification you use to back your claims should be realistic, convincing, and well supported. What guarantees do you offer?

Fill in the blanks with the way you want your practice to fit into your local market.

To _____ (name target patients) _____ (name of your practice) _____ is a _____ (category in which you want to be considered) that delivers _____ (the unique service you want patients to associate with your practice not already taken by any competitors) because _____ (explanation of why they should trust your claims) _____

_____

_____

**Example**

To (Medicare recipients):

Elder Eye Care Group is a geriatric-oriented ophthalmic practice that prides itself on delivering specialized low-vision services and visual assistance for the partially sighted and visually impaired. Our providers are both residency and specialty trained with 20 years' experience serving the community.

## Notes

1. Deutsch B. Charting a course with strategic marketing. *Bank Marketing*. September 1998;30(9):28–34.
2. Piirto R. Measuring minds in the 1990s. *American Demographics*. December 1990;12(12):30(6).
3. Perrault W, McCarthy E. *Basic Marketing*. Boston: Irwin McGraw-Hill; 1999:79.
4. Modified from Your marketing plan. AOA Practice Enhancement Program II, precourse workbook. St. Louis, MO: American Optometric Association; 1986.
5. Kotler P, Clarke R. *Marketing for Healthcare Organizations*. Englewood Cliffs, NJ: Prentice-Hall; 1987:244.
6. Adapted from Selbert. *U.S. News & World Report*. 1995:3.
7. Engelberg M, Neubrand S. Building sensible segmentation strategies in managed care. *Marketing Health Services*. Summer 1997;17(2):50.
8. Girish P, Stewart D. Cluster analysis in marketing research. *Journal of Marketing Research*. May 1983:134–148.
9. Dietz J. When Gen X meets aging Baby Boomers. *Marketing News*. May 10, 1999:17–18.
10. Generation Y. *Business Week*. February 15, 1999:80–83.
11. Kanzler F. The positioning statement: Have one before you start communicating. *Public Relations Quarterly*. Winter 1997–1998:18–20.
12. Ries A, Trout J. *Positioning: The Battle for Your Mind*. New York: Warner Books; 1981.
13. Berry L, Lefkowith E, Clark T. In services, what's in a name? *Harvard Business Review*. September–October 1988:28–30.
14. Modified from Sturm A. *The New Rules of Healthcare Marketing*. Chicago: Health Administration Press; 1998:17.
15. McGoldrick T, Hyatt D, Laflin L. How big is big enough? *Marketing Tools*. May 1998:54–58.
16. Alreck P, Settle R. *The Survey Research Handbook*. Boston: McGraw-Hill; 1995.

# CHAPTER 5

# Building Long-Term Patient Relationships

You were born an original, don't die a copy.

—*John Mason*

## The Value of Patient Retention

The relationships formed between patients, provider, and practice staff are possibly the most valuable asset to the successful longevity of a practice. The tactics an ECP uses to acquire, establish, and retain patients have come to be known as *relationship marketing*. Creating long-term customer relationships is the cornerstone and goal of every successful service-oriented business. In addition, the most valuable patient is one that offers greater potential revenue and profit by returning more often and exhibiting greater loyalty. Consumer research released in 1994, entitled "Measured Marketing," found that the top 30% of customers contribute 70% of revenue, while the bottom 30% contribute just 3%.[1] These "select" patients from the top group are more likely to recommend your practice to others, cost less to maintain, and are willing to pay premium fees, recognizing the benefits your services offer. Don't ignore the bottom 30% because they are not select patients, but spend the majority of your marketing efforts aimed at those patients most likely to support your practice.

A tangible way to realize the value of long-term patient retention is to calculate the present value of keeping a patient for a period of years. As an example, take a patient who spends $300

**Table 5–1    Calculating the Present Value of the Lifetime Worth of a Patient**

| | Today | Year 1 | Year 2 | Year 20 | Total Value |
|---|---|---|---|---|---|
| PV @ 8% risk rate | $= \$300 +$ | $\dfrac{300(1.05)^1}{1.08^1} +$ | $\dfrac{300(1.05)^2}{1.08^2} + \ldots +$ | $\dfrac{300(1.05)^{20}}{1.08^{20}}$ | $= \$4,652$ |
| PV @ 14% risk rate | $= \$300 +$ | $\dfrac{300(1.05)^1}{1.14^1} +$ | $\dfrac{300(1.05)^2}{1.14^2} + \ldots +$ | $\dfrac{300(1.05)^{20}}{1.14^{20}}$ | $= \$3,067$ |

per year in your office, assume a 5% annual increase in fee, a 20-year period, and two different risk (discount) rates (one very safe, equivalent to the U.S. Government Fund Index of 8%, the other of moderate risk, equivalent to the past 20-year average annual return rate of 14% for equity mutual funds).[2] By simply performing a present value calculation as shown in Table 5–1, the lifetime (20-year) value of a patient at the minimum is worth between $3,000 and $4,600 equivalent value in today's dollar to the ECP's practice. By the way, General Motors estimates the lifetime value of a loyal Cadillac customer is $332,000, and at Pizza Hut, a lifetime customer is worth $8,000.[3]

One way to obtain "patients for life" is to begin when they are infants, the belief of W. David Sullins, Jr., OD, FAAO of Athens, Tennessee, past president of the AOA, who states:

> the best way we found to build our practice was having a special interest in children. Interestingly enough, we are now restating and recommitting that interest in a new concept in infant eye care for the new millennium. The program is called Operation Bright Start. We learned that nationally, there were 86% of our children that received no eye care of any kind as they entered the first grade. We have agreed to provide eye care to infants in their first year of life without charge for our services. As in the past, we know that taking proper care of the mother's or grandmother's infant will be the best introduction to our philosophy of eye care. We feel we must introduce parents and grandparents to eye care as a most important part of infant and child development. We now know that once a patient has entrusted their most important asset with us we have an obligation to remain state of the art in knowledge, instrumentation, physical plant,

staffing and convenience. Our experience has been that the parents and grandparents follow the lead of their infants and children.[4]

The intangible nature of the eyecare service business, with high levels of provider-patient interaction, offers an ECP a greater opportunity to develop customer loyalty than a primarily product-oriented business.[5] The ECP has the advantage of providing patients a nearly unknown, constantly changing service encounter that offers patients the opportunity to experience provider performance that can greatly influence their perceptions.[6] A recently conducted public opinion poll revealed that recommendations of family and friends were the number one reason why patients chose health care providers.[7]

## ECP-Patient Marketing Bonds

An ECP can develop three levels of bonding with patients through the implementation of a marketing program.[8] Level one, referred to as *frequency* or *retention marketing*, uses only financial incentive to strengthen the relationship. This is achieved primarily through price cutting, such as special short-term sales or the buy-one-get-one-free tactic, as the method of coercing patients to spend more. These tactics may become problematic because typically they offer only limited short-term advantages over the competition. The result may be a temporary period of increased volume and gross revenue, possibly accompanied by decreased marginal profit. **Lowering prices is the easiest of the marketing mix strategies for a competitor to copy, and price alone does not offer the ECP sustained advantages.**

A more-developed, level two relationship adds a social bond by personalizing patient communications and stressing the concept of the "patient as a person" rather than a blanket marketing of a uniform message to all patients. Marketing tactics commonly emphasize staying in touch with patients through various communication media and learning the specific needs of targeted groups. Two-way communication strengthens patient perceptions about their relationship with an ECP, especially if the patient is not always the one to initiate contact. Once this level of relationship has been established, it offers the ECP a small cushion of patient forgiveness if a service failure should occur, at least to the point where patients will allow the ECP's office the opportunity to rectify errors before abandoning the office.[7]

The highest-level relationship is characterized by a structural bond formed as an integral component of the service delivery process as opposed to evolving from practice personnel relationships or choice of business strategies. Level three structural bonds are achieved by providing patients with services not offered by competitors; often, this is technology related, such as the latest examining equipment, because this is a continually changing area that can be upgraded by ECPs. Internet and database marketing are two recent advances that can be considered level three relationship enhancements to bolster the doctor-patient relationship. **Marketing to patients "as a segment of one" is a new concept, made possible by the abilities of databases and the Internet.** First, patients must have access to the Internet and initiate contact when their needs originate. Market your website URL and e-mail address every chance you have. An ECP can enhance this aspect of relationship building by sending out occasional Internet communications or newsletters. This also allows the ECP to thank patients for their continued patronage. A management database system that allows the ECP to customize communications to each patient is another enhancement enabled by advances in technology. "The key to level three marketing is to provide *value-adding services* . . . that are not readily available elsewhere."[9] **For the eyecare setting, ocular health e-letters, on-line illustrated eyewear, and contact lens ordering are all forms of level three marketing that could offer competitive advantages in the near future.**

## Relationship Marketing

Marketing evolved, starting in the 1950s, from a transaction-centered process concerned with short-term, single-sale customer encounters to, in the 1970s, a focus on marketing products to society.[10] In the 1980s, attention shifted to marketing the services a business can offer. Relationship marketing is the culmination of this progression that recognizes two market forces.[9] First, marketing must "anticipate and attend to an expanse of sectors including customer markets, supply markets, internal markets, referral markets and influencer markets."[10] Second, constantly changing patient needs and external market forces (economy, third party, and regulatory agencies) require the ECP to possess a thorough understanding and acceptance of the components of relationship marketing.

Much of traditional and current eyecare marketing concerns "getting" patients. This limited view of marketing implies that the ECP's primary role is to get the right product to the right patient at the right time "by perceiving, understanding, stimulating and satisfying the needs of specially selected target markets."[10] Relationship marketing takes the concept further, with the addition of "keeping" patients as an objective. This requires the ECP to take a much broader view of all the factors that affect the perception of value that patients make about the ECP's products and services. The "six markets" model shown in Figure 5–1 suggests several different sources for which the ECP must develop different strategies and activities, including current and potential patients, employees, agencies, referral sources, and suppliers.

The primary emphasis of marketing should be directed at the patient, however, many practices direct the majority of their attention toward attracting new patients at the expense of fostering heightened relationships with current patients. The risk of this strategy is known as the *leaking bucket effect*, where current

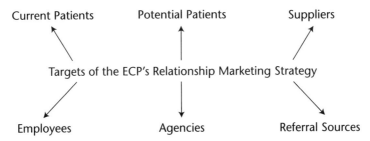

**Figure 5–1    Targets of ECP's relationship marketing strategy. (Modified from Christopher M, Payne A, Ballantyne D.** *Relationship Marketing.* **Oxford: Butterworth–Heinemann; 1996:21.)**

patients abandon the practice due to inadequate, ongoing communication with the ECP's practice.[9]

It is difficult to dispute that word-of-mouth promotion by a satisfied patient is by far the most cost-effective method to gain referrals for your practice. But satisfied patients are not the only referral source you can cultivate. Consider what formal relationships can be established with referral sources such as PCPs, corporate personnel managers, and school administrators. These sources act as intermediaries and can be third parties, agencies, or networks. In eyecare today, as in many other industries, these intermediaries have two things in common: Their significance in referring patients is becoming greater and there are more of them.[9] The cost and benefit to your practice of developing a relationship marketing strategy for these referral sources should be determined. Benefits from relationships with these intermediaries often take awhile to realize. Jennifer Mallinger, O.D., and Chen Young, O.D., of Las Vegas, NV, were surprised to find out that the private preschools and elementary schools in their area did not have school nurses to provide school screenings. To market their new practice, they "called up the school principals, made up permission slips for the parents, and arranged for a date to perform vision screenings. We gave all the teachers copies of the reports to give to the parents and we received many responses. We now have not only these students as our patients, but their families as well. We have become the community optometrists."[11]

The relationships you develop through membership in community organizations can be a tremendous source of referral, especially after you have contributed time and established an image as a member who gives to the community. In the words of Mort Silverman, public health and practice management instructor at Nova University in Florida, referral from civic groups was

> one area that I felt made a major contribution to building my practice. I opened cold turkey in a new suburban community with no local ties what-so-ever. For the next two years, I was out six nights a week participating in the Grange, Masons, "Hoxsie" Community Club, Junior Chamber of Commerce, became a scoutmaster, . . . and every other organization that I could find the time for. It eventually paid off.[12]

Supplier relationships have changed from the traditional adversarial model to one based on cooperation directed at achieving maximum benefit for both parties. No longer should securing the best price from suppliers be the top priority. This strategy often results in unpredictable deliveries and inferior goods, more often from wholesale labs but at times from manufacturers. Alliances with suppliers, often overlooked, is an area to which to pay attention, while developing a specific relationship marketing strategy. The largest single area of expense in an ECP's practice is the supplies. Most ECP offices spend between 25 and 40% of their total revenue on goods and services purchased from outside suppliers. This compares to 60% spent by U.S. manufacturers.[13]

Support of the value of vendor partnerships is mounting, as evidenced by a study in the electronics industry, which revealed firms that formed supplier alliances outperformed firms that had not formed alliances.[14] According to Dr. Michael Spitzer of Irvine, California, "my secret to success is to let your reps know that you will try anything to see if it works. Be open-minded about new things, give them a try, and if it works use it more. Reps will appreciate this and always contact you when something new hits."[15] The ECP should develop strong affiliations with suppliers through their marketing efforts. This can be achieved by forming comarketing or vendor partnerships fundamental to "the concept of both parties agreeing and as a result creating a better future for each other."[9]

Arguably the number 1 complaint by ECPs today is obtaining competent, loyal staff members, a trend that will continue to afflict the eyecare industry for many years. One way for the ECP to respond is to develop a specific relationship marketing strategy to compete in the increasingly competitive employee pool. Periodically, place classifieds for positions in your office and assemble resumés to stay abreast of your current market. In the words of Dr. Denise Howard, Bloomington, Indiana, "my success has been a result of my investment in a great staff and up-to-date technology. I hire the friendliest, nicest people I can find even if they have no health care or optical experience. Skills can be learned but personalities cannot be altered much."[16]

Employee relationship marketing encompasses two perspectives. First, personal selling by the ECP promoting practice objectives; second, external marketing of job opportunities to potential employees. During periods of high unemployment, adequate clerical personnel will likely be available; the demographics of younger workers reveal that it is crucial for ECPs to develop a specific employee relationship marketing strategy, especially during better economic periods.[17]

The final relationship marketing targets for the ECP are agencies, which refer to the government and regulatory bodies that empower and limit the boundaries of an ECP practice. This type of marketing, typically performed as public relations or lobbying, usually is most effective when performed as an organized group. However, a well-formulated, specific, and comprehensive relationship marketing strategy often is performed on a reactive basis, rather than the more effective ongoing proactive basis.[18]

Relationship marketing suggests that the ECP would benefit by developing enhanced relationships with not only patients but employees, suppliers, referral sources, and agencies affecting ECP practices; however, it probably is unnecessary to create a formal relationship strategy plan for all sectors. The bonds you form with each of these sectors through a relationship marketing strategy ultimately influence your ability to deliver the quality and value necessary to create and retain a loyal patient base.

## Creating Value Through a Brand

Successful relationship marketing requires adequate effort in creating value for patients. Patients have different concepts and beliefs as to what gives them value. When choosing eyecare services, patients will be attracted to one of three groups:[19] practices that provide low prices and convenience, practices that embellish services offering strong one-to-one relationships, and practices that use the latest technological equipment and highest quality products. Price is only one part of the total experience that allows the patient to form the overall perception of value received at your practice. Given that value equals quality divided by cost ($V = Q/C$), it follows that the three levels of the doctor-patient bond suggest that low price is not the only way to produce high value. The perception of customer service, which is an integral component of the value patients believe they receive, can vary greatly, ranging from timely and reliable delivery of products and services to all the activities, communication, and follow-up your practice performs to ensure what you promise to deliver meets your patient's expectations.[20] Another popular view of customer service adds an "understanding of what the customer buys and determining how additional value can be added to the product or service being offered."[9] The perception of value can be enhanced through the creation of a practice brand; however, "one of the important elements that sets a brand name apart from others is that it carries an inherent promise that the branded item is of greater value or outperforms the non–brand-name."[21]

### Building Loyalty Through a Practice Brand

A brand is the "trust" you create between your patients and your practice enhanced by the actions of you and your staff. **The ECP's practice brand comprises the sum of the patient's experience and features you and your staff provide to create a distinct, memorable identity of your practice in the patient's mind.** A brand consists of such primary practice components as pricing policies, quality of service and products dispensed, staff interaction with patients, and the overall appearance of the office and equipment. The value of a brand is how successfully you can differentiate your services from the competition. A brand can be enhanced by a name, logo, slogan, or any other mechanism you use to provide patients the opportunity to distinguish your practice from others. The practice brand is considered the principal brand, producing the greatest impact on your services, as opposed to a product brand, which is the primary brand for goods. **A brand is transmitted to patients through various media, including signs, print (brochures, letterhead, newsletters), visual symbols, staff uniforms, and mass media.** However, the brand you want to project is not always guaranteed to be what the patient perceives. The message you want your practice brand to convey must be uniform and pervasive throughout all media used. If not, your patients may have conflicting perceptions.

The meaning the patient perceives from the brand is what influences his or her impression, the ultimate classification of the ECP's practice. What you want your practice to represent becomes the "promise" you intend to deliver to your patients. To gain the most benefit from a brand identity, this promise should be valued highly by patients, unique from your competitors, believable, and compatible with your practice's capabilities and strengths.[22]

> Brand meaning is a function of brand presentation and service concept, quality and value. The service the company provides, how well it performs the service, and the service's value combine to influence the customer's interpretation of the presented brand. Its principal role is to give the firm a marketing edge by reinforcing the firm's service in a way that is differentiating, important and commanding to customers.[9]

External conditions in the ECP's marketplace favor the use of a brand, several of which are listed in Table 5–2.

### Creating Your Practice Brand

The first step in building a strong brand identity starts with research based on patient focus groups and industrywide obser-

---

**Table 5–2  Market Conditions That Favor the Use of a Brand**

---

1. You are in a local marketplace where patients might perceive your services to be similar in quality and value to the competition.

2. When appealing to new patients that have no experience with any of the competitors in a local area, a strong brand may have better success in attracting patients.

3. Your brand is well known and established for one type of service (such as contact lens specialist) and you want to extend that favorable perception to a new service you wish to offer (such as low vision).

4. If you decide to change your strategy, you can piggyback a new brand onto an already established brand (such as when bringing in an associate).

5. If you want to establish barriers to protect your existing volume and level of revenue from competitive encroachment, a study conducted by Chris Easingwood* found that reputation and brand were the two most-effective methods of deterring innovative techniques by competitors.

---

*Easingwood C. Service design and service company strategy. In: *Marketing Operations, Human Resources and Insights into Services*. France: University of Marseilles; 1990:188–199.

**Table 5–3  Questions to Create a Brand Identity**

1. What makes a difference to patients in selecting an ECP?
2. How do patients compare ECPs?
3. What is most important to patients about obtaining eye care?
4. What eye care benefits do patients value most?

Adapted from Arpin D. Medical group marketing: Is your group a brand name? *Marketer's Guidepost*. September–October 1997;8(4):2.

vations on the use of brand meaning. Creating a brand identity starts by finding the answers to the questions concerning patient needs found in Table 5–3. If you decide to change or augment the direction of your business strategy, use the existing brand rather than create a new one to jump-start the new service and product offerings. Involve your staff in development and training to reinforce the goals of the ECP brand.

A patient may experience your practice brand in many different ways before, during, and after the actual encounter. All these influence points offer an opportunity to monitor and enhance the patient's perception about the brand image. Prior to any visit, word of mouth and referral sources that have been properly capitalized on can offer positive reinforcement. During the visit, the ease and comfort the practice offers the patient, the interaction with the ECP and staff, and the physical condition of the practice surroundings and equipment all have a direct bearing on the patient's perception of your practice brand. Finally, after the visit, you can solidify your brand image through the ease of the patient's billing insurance policies and the quality of communication with the patient. A brand identity that is desirable to develop in many industries is ETDBW, which is an acronym for *easy to do business with*,[23] examples of which include evening, early morning, and weekend appointments, and financing.

**The Practice Brand Name**

The brand name is by far the most important aspect of creating a brand identity. While sometimes only a graphic image or symbol, it establishes a perceived or invented reputation with patients that can offer business advantages in highly competitive markets.[24]

Choose a brand name that is easily presented in a variety of innovative ways, using different media. The following five characteristics contribute to an ECP's brand by increasing patient awareness and recognition:[25]

1. *Distinctiveness.* Does your brand distinguish you from the competition immediately?
2. *Relevance.* Is it easy for patients to recognize the benefits you offer and nature of your business?
3. *Memorability.* Is it easy for your name to be recalled, used, and understood?
4. *Flexibility.* In how many different formats, medias, and strategies can the brand be used?
5. *Legality.* Is it defendable from another company claiming rights to the name?

Lenscrafters is an example of an eyecare business that successfully adapted these five qualities into the development of a brand through their slogan, Eyeglasses in an Hour. Distinctiveness (and legality) is achieved through onsite surfacing labs with the ability to make glasses in 1 hour. Consumers perceive relevance through the personal convenience of time savings. The variety of print, direct mail, newspaper, radio, magazine, and television promotion increases memorability by maintaining consumer contact and has proven to be flexible in its longevity of use in all the different media. A similar analysis can be made of Wal-Mart's brand (always the lowest price), Ritz Carlton Hotels (superior quality), and Nordstrom (customer service).

One factor driving the increase in the use of brands and advertising in all sectors of the health care industry is the maturing of the managed care industry in many locations. A major source of new patients for any provider is the result of a shift away from the competition.[26] This can be facilitated through the use of a brand identity. It is recommended that a brand name be brief and simple. One method of achieving a unique name is to use words not usually associated with eyecare business or the ophthalmic industry, proper names or fabricated names. A patient's ability to identify your brand and the position you wish to occupy in your local area marketplace is enhanced by a brand name that conveys the nature of your practice and the benefits you offer. As an example, Humana, the large West Coast health care organization, chose a name that connotes caring sensitive service, an especially positive image to convey for a health care company. Do not use terms that might limit patient perceptions about your services unless you are offering limited service and product choices, as with a practice limited to a single specialty.[9]

### Using a Brand to Enhance Practice Identity

A major goal of image development is to determine how you want your patients to perceive your practice. One way to achieve this is to help patients comprehend the value your practice offers relative to your competitors. This originates with your practice mission and is conveyed through the values you uphold. Appendix 5–1 is used by practitioners to determine what identity they are conveying to their patients; it can be useful with staff members as well. Do your staff members know for what you stand? Do they know what identity you wish to convey to the patients? Ask staff members to select terms according to what they would like to see as the perfect office. Have them answer the question, Which of these attributes do you wish would describe the office in which you work? You may be surprised by their attitudes. Then, ask yourself, Which of the attributes best describes the way you are with your patients and your staff? You may learn that you must make changes in yourself before you can begin to change the practice identity. Your marketing techniques must be consistent with your practice identity or you will lose credibility. Losing credibility with your patients will cause you to lose business faster than if you didn't market at all.

How does your image affect your day-to-day responsibilities? The practice brand concept is where to start making decisions about the image you want to develop. As the owner, everything that occurs in the practice is your responsibility. A good way to begin making decisions is to examine the effect of your decision on the marketability of your practice image. Remember that marketing is supposed to create a desire to buy products and services.

Keep this in mind. Focus your efforts on this goal. You can find many examples of marketing that do not instill a desire to buy anything, such as an obvious hard sell or a noninformative, noncaring salesperson.

Marketing can be thought of as the truth made interesting and communicated to target populations. To maintain your credibility, you must communicate the truth about yourself. Who are you and what image do you convey? Some say image is what we do, the way the public sees us, whether true or not, or a combination of the two. Others say image is nothing more than advertisement, public relations, and promotion.

What image do you see when you think of an employee of the CIA? The CIA agent is dressed in a dark conservative suit and a white long-sleeved shirt with a black tie. They wear black socks above perfectly polished black wing tips. Their hair is cut short and neatly trimmed. The movie *Men in Black* used this image with their characters because it is consistent with what we expect from federal government policing agencies. Now contrast this image with what comes to mind for a representative of the U.S. Postal Service? In the 1980s, it would have been Cliff, the character on the television show *Cheers*, with white socks, black shoes, and a short sleeve gray-blue post office uniform. In the early 1990s, it would be Newman, the neighbor from *Seinfeld*. What do you think of when you think of an eye doctor? Usually a conservative appearing man or woman wearing a white coat and . . . glasses.

Is image just appearance? Is image a symbol, sign, ad, logo? The CIA logo says strong, high tech, stable, modern. What is the U.S. Postal Service logo? Previously it was an eagle in flight, yet we knew the postal service was inefficient and slow. Promos and logos are not effective unless they deliver the type of products and service promised, such as reliable, dependable, fashionable, or expedient eyecare. These are essential components of developing a practice brand of excellence.

Your image actually is determined by the patient's total interaction with your practice. This explains how one ECP can build a practice through community interaction while another cannot. You can only build your practice if you maintain the image a patient expects of an eye doctor during all interactions with the community. The successful ECP will take the time to learn what qualities will enhance a practice image. One way to obtain this knowledge is through patient surveys and focus group discussions. You must fit the patient's idea of an eye doctor by conveying a professional image through your practice brand, or you will lose potential patients.

When you communicate your true practice identity by marketing your practice brand, the public perceives you as you represent yourself; this generates confidence. A main reason patients choose an office is confidence in that office. Don't be the old eagle of the post office. Convey your identity through your practice brand in all aspects of marketing. Convey your identity in all decisions you make concerning your practice. If you want an identity associated with eyecare (a service) as opposed to eyewear (a product), good communication is paramount; do this by making the office visit enjoyable for your patients. Patients are not necessarily able to judge the accuracy or quality of the clinical care they receive; however, they definitely judge the care you deliver on aspects they can understand: ease of obtaining an appointment, receptionist's phone demeanor and greeting, reception room cleanliness, and fee misunderstandings. There's an old saying, "never go to a doctor with dead plants." If he or she can't take care of plants, how will he or she take care of patients? Your prospective patients don't know you, your office, your products, or your services—except for what they learn from the way you convey your marketing and how they perceive your practice brand. Clarifying your practice brand in their mind will avoid any contradictions that may develop about your identity.

To win their patronage, you have to prove yourself stable, successful, and confident. The idea is for you to remain consistent. Be consistent in your theme, your format, your graphics, your media, your identity. Give them something positive to count on. Your patients will feel comfort, security, and safety in the consistency of your message. If they want anything from a new venture, it's the assurance that they won't go wrong if they choose your services. The more you remain consistent with your practice decisions, the more assured they will be. Be consistent in conveying your identity.[27] Appendix 5–1 will help you determine your present practice brand identity as well as those qualities you may wish to be recognized by your patients.

### Using a Logo

A logo is another marketing tactic used to reinforce awareness and convey a message about quality. The fastest growing segment of the advertising industry is corporate giveaways, such as pens and mugs, that only have the company logo.[28] A logo should be recognizable, familiar, evoke a common meaning to the target consumer, and produce a positive result.[29] Logos are considered the best way to advertise in the Yellow Pages.[30] Research on logo recognition indicates that, to achieve maximum effectiveness and recognition, the design should be slightly elaborate, meaningfully natural, and harmonious with respect to symmetry and balance.[31] If you decide to use a logo, ask yourself what characteristics of design will create the response you desire. Consumers must be able to correctly recognize a logo, then recall the business name or brand. Make sure it conveys the brand image you are developing. When developing a logo, seek answers to the following questions from staff and patients that know the type of practice you want to develop:[32]

1. Is the logo visually appealing?
2. Is the message that it sends about this practice innovative?
3. Will patients understand it?
4. Would it motivate a patient to read a mailing or newspaper item?
5. Does it inspire confidence in the abilities of this practice?

## Moment of Truth Analysis

A major goal of developing your practice brand identity is to determine how you want your patients to perceive your practice. One way to achieve this is to make patients comprehend the value your practice offers relative to your competitors. This originates with your practice mission and is conveyed through values you uphold. One concept you can use to help make your practice uniquely different is to adapt a "moment of truth" analysis suggested in the late 1980s by Jan Carlzon, former CEO of Scandinavian Airlines.[33]

The moment of truth concept describes critical encounter points within a practice that can sway the impression a patient forms. These moments are neither good nor bad but manageable in your favor should you actively identify and define what you would like the ideal outcome to be for the patient. The goal of defining each moment of truth encounter is to create a positive impact on the patient. This is accomplished by creating service standards for every interaction a patient has with practice personnel that may have the potential to affect patient loyalty, retention, and referrals. You also can develop enhanced levels of service strategy through the "service mapping" process by using a "process flow diagram" for all of a patient's significant contact points with personnel.[34]

Start by analyzing the patient office visit cycle from start to finish. This sequence of events begins when the patient first calls the office for an appointment. What is the attitude of your staff on the telephone? Does your receptionist make a positive first impression by being kind, sincere, helpful, and friendly? How long before the phone typically is answered? For how long are callers put on hold? An analysis can be performed by keeping track of the subject matter of calls and which portions of your operations are receiving what percentage of calls. It is possible to make this area more efficient by changing the demand.[35] As an example, if you find that your office receives an inordinate number of calls from patients waiting for glasses or contact lenses, you might find it would save the staff or patient time by sending patients postcards or phoning them when products are ready.

On entering the office, does your staff greet a patient within 30 seconds or does a patient wait 2–4 minutes at the front desk before being acknowledged? Do your staff create a caring atmosphere by addressing the patient by name? How patient-friendly is your reception area? Are all the office policies and forms fully explained to avoid possible misunderstanding about the amount of insurance benefit coverage to which the patient is entitled?

Take advantage of the patient's time in the patient lounge (not waiting room) by making it part of the experience to achieve your marketing goals. Present visual and multimedia messages while the patient is waiting. Emergency room patients at Robert Wood Johnson University Hospital in New Brunswick, NJ, are given this guarantee: patients not seen by a nurse within 15 minutes or a doctor within 30 minutes are given *free* care. Is the patient lounge spotless, modern, and regularly monitored, with appropriate reading materials and informative signs pertaining to patient well-being? After the patient is escorted to the exam room, is infection control emphasized by the staff member wiping down surfaces with a disinfectant? If the wait is going to be for several minutes, are there reading materials for the patient if pretesting has been completed? When the eyecare provider enters the exam room, is hand washing the first thing done in view of the patient to reinforce the infection control concept? On completion of the all important case summary presentation, are the account settlement procedures explained? Prior to leaving is the patient given a specific date for a reappointment with a proper explanation? The ideal patient visit is a model all ECPs should strive to develop and continually upgrade in their practice. Portions of a sample ideal patient visit are described in Table 5–4 should the reader decide to undertake a "moment of truth" analysis.

Several significant moments of truth occur during the patient encounter. One is the transition that occurs after the ECP has presented the patient with the case findings, made recommendations, and turns the patient over to a staff member to dispense the eyewear. Here, the patient encounter transforms from a service-oriented to a product-oriented experience, a moment of truth that could result in negative consequences to the practice and its revenue if not handled properly. At this point, the ECP loses direct contact with the patient and there will be great opportunity for patient indecision.

## Patient Routing Slip

Take the time during the postexam case summary to explain the advantages of various options, such as antireflective coating or ultraviolet protection. However, patients with little background in eyecare may not fully understand nor remember all the ECP's

**Table 5–4    Ideal Patient Visit**

I. Making the Appointment
1. Staff member responding to call is courteous, thorough, attentive, respectful, and accommodating.
2. Patient is addressed by name and given an appropriately timed appointment, based on urgency and patient's needs.

II. Checking in at Reception
1. Patient is greeted promptly upon arrival.
2. Appropriate paperwork is completed and patient is advised of benefit entitlements.
3. Patient waits a reasonable time in patient lounge with adequate, entertaining, ambient surroundings.

III. Exam
1. Staff member introduces himself or herself and escorts patient to exam room, seats patient, and gives preliminary tests or instructions.
2. After exam, the provider offers a diagnosis, options, and makes and justifies recommendations. Patient is told how and when to perform the next step.
3. Any opportunities for preventive eyecare are discussed, and patient is encouraged to ask any additional unanswered questions.

IV. Checking Out
1. Follow-up appointments and referrals are made, including an explanation of why further care is needed.
2. Payment is arranged, with an explanation of benefits applied toward total fee.

Modified from *Patient Satisfaction and Outcomes Measurement*. Washington, DC: Internal Medicine Center for Advance Research and Education; January 1998:9.

recommendations by the time they get to the dispensary. One way to augment and bolster the ECP's influence over product sales is to use a patient routing slip as a written form of instruction to staff assisting patients. Staff members may have no way of knowing what specific recommendations the ECP has made to the patient regarding the selection of eyeglasses or contact lenses. Dispensary personnel may be hesitant to make recommendations to patients without the ECP's instructions or approval. Even if they do, recommendations from office staff, no matter how knowledgeable, seldom have the same weight in the minds of patients as recommendations from the ECP. The use of a routing slip will enhance the continual flow of the patient through this phase of the visit. It also provides the staff member with direct guidance as to what should be offered to the patient. A sample patient routing slip is shown in Figure 5–2.

With growing patient volume a reality (and a necessity) in most practices, ECPs have little time to assist staff members, reassure patients, and make recommendations regarding eyewear. However, the information gap that sometimes occurs when the practitioner turns the patient over to the dispensary staff can result in the patient not getting the eyewear that really is needed. It also can have a negative impact with regard to practice revenue.

The routing slip commonly is used in many businesses to assure orders are processed smoothly and efficiently. The technique easily is adapted to eyecare practice as a way to help ensure that the practitioner's recommendations to the patient are incorporated into the eyewear dispensed. Routing slips are preprinted forms with spaces provided to check off or fill in routinely required information. The format should be designed to quickly convey the specific information needed to do a job efficiently and effectively. The ECP easily can fill out the form while conferring with the patient during the postexamination and hand it to a staff member as the patient enters the dispensary.

An eyecare practice routing slip can provide an easy, effective way to convey information on the exact spectacles or contact lenses recommended by the practitioner or the care required for the patient. The practitioner simply fills out the routing slip during the postexamination consultation with the patient and hands the slip to the dispensary staff person. The slip can be used to designate the exact brand and type (disposable, daily wear, extended wear, toric, gas permeable) of contact lens to be dispensed or the brand and type (single vision, bifocal, PAL, high index, polycarbonate) of spectacle lenses to be dispensed along with the recommended add-ons such as UV protection or antiglare coating.

The form, as shown in Figure 5–2, can help staff members efficiently schedule patients for follow-up care, such as dilated fundus examinations, visual fields, or contact lens fittings and can ensure patients are referred for necessary care, specifying the

I. Follow-up care:

DFE _____

VF _____

　　　Screening _____ Threshold _____

　　Referral to _____ for _____

　　Progress Evaluation _____

　　　　　Contact lens fit/problem _____

　　　　　　　Trial lens given _____

　　　　　　　Trial lens to order _____

　　　　TPA Tx _____

II. Spectacles lens type to purchase:

SV _____

Bif _____ Type _____

PAL _____ Brand _____

A/R _____ UV _____

Hi Index _____ Polycarb _____

III. Contact lens type to purchase:

Disposable _____ Brand _____

　　　3 mo. ____ 6 mo. ____ 12 mo. ____ Other ____

Daily wear soft _____ Brand _____

Extended wear _____ Brand _____

Toric _____ Brand _____

Gas Perm _____ Brand _____

\- - - - - - - - - - - - - - - - - - - - - - - - - - - - - - - - - - - - - - - - - - - - - -

**For office use only (coded to prevent patient awareness)**

\- - - - - - - - - - - - - - - - - - - - - - - - - - - - - - - - - - - - - - - - - - - - - -

**Capture Rate**

Patient did purchase ____

　　Type of product _____ Brand _____

Patient did not purchase ____

　　Reason given by patient _____

　　Reason staff member suspects _____

**Figure 5–2　Patient routing slip.**

condition diagnosed and the doctor to whom the patient is referred. For ECPs, routing slips represent an easy, efficient communication tool. For staff members, the slip provides direct guidance on what should be offered the patient conveying the practitioner's authority. The routing slip provides a means through which a staff member can reinforce the ECP's recommendations by addressing the patient with comments such as, "Well now, Mrs. Smith, the doctor recommends that you have ultraviolet protection in your spectacle lenses" or "the doctor recommends you be scheduled for a visual field examination." It also can provide an important means of measuring exactly how often patients actually choose the correction recommended by the practitioner.

The second section of the routing slip, for office use only, should be used to record the type and brand of lenses the practitioner actually purchased, as opposed to those recommended by the practitioner, or to note if the patient purchased nothing. Patient comments can be noted. This section, coded to be interpreted only by office staff, can be a valuable source of practice management information. On the basis of this section, sales results can be tabulated by staff to provide a figure known in marketing as the *capture rate*. The number of patients complying with the ECP's recommendations can be documented; the percentage choosing various lens options and features can be tracked; and trends can be monitored. ECPs can identify what products are enjoying more success than others and what percentage of patients are not buying specifically recommended items and for what reasons. Based on that information, ECPs may decide to change marketing strategies or pricing policies for specific products. The data also can indicate which office personnel have highest capture rates. ECPs can offer training to those with lower success rates. As a communications aid for the ECP and source of practice management guidance for the staff, patient routing slips should be used in more eyecare practices in the future. However, the greatest benefits ultimately may be realized by patients, for whom routing slips provide greater assurance that they will get the care and correction they require.

## Reasons Patients May Leave Your Practice

Choose policies and procedures that are consistent with your identity. In every decision you make regarding your practice, devote your attention to excellence, that is what patients want. Not offering excellence will speed the demise of your office, and marketing that is inaccurate or dishonest will cause you to fail even faster. It is unfortunate in many instances, but word-of-mouth promotion about poor quality spreads faster than praise for good quality. Research about why consumers stop using the services of a business shows:[36]

3% move from the area.
9% choose the competition.
14% are dissatisfied with the products provided.
68% cite an attitude of not caring about the customer by either the
    owner or an employee.

Appendix 5–2 shows the ECP how to analyze the reasons patients may leave your office.

    Use the table in Appendix 5–3 to evaluate each opportunity you have to communicate your image to your patients. Determine whether a particular tactic needs improvement in your practice. The table may help you conclude that you have been ignoring many opportunities to communicate your image to your patients or that you have been communicating an inconsistent image to your patients. Use this to add to your overall marketing strategy. Appendices 5–2 and 5–3 will assist you in analyzing the specific strengths, weaknesses, and needs of present marketing tactics. Additional tactics will be discussed in detail in the next chapter as part of the discussion on how to best manage the marketing mix.

> The customer isn't always right. However, the customer is always the customer, and I want the customer to always be mine.
> —*John Hartley, Promus Hotel Corporation,*
> *in "Best Practices in Customer Service"*

## Action Plan for ECPs

1. Use the Practice Brand Identity exercise (Appendix 5–1) to determine the following three items:
   a. The present image you and your staff believe you project.
   b. The image your patients believe you project.
   c. The image you and your staff wish to project.
2. Complete Appendix 5–2, Reasons Patients Leave Your Practice, to determine what changes you may wish to make.
3. Perform a start to finish moment of truth analysis to identify patient encounter points you wish to change.
4. Review the Marketing During the Patient Visit (Appendix 5–3) to identify the various marketing methods you can use to enhance your desired brand image.
5. Inform and educate your staff about these desired changes.
6. Seek input and train staff on the best ways to initiate changes.

# Practice Brand Identity

Look over the following list of attributes. Circle those that best describe your eyecare practitioner's office. Asterisk those that you wish described your eyecare practitioner's office.

| | | |
|---|---|---|
| Caring | Fashionable | Aloof |
| High tech | Inexpensive | Indifferent |
| Up on most recent information | Convenient | Traditional |
| A leader in the profession | Fast | Trendy |
| Old fashioned | Comprehensive | Laid back |
| Fun | Child oriented | Flashy |
| Good-natured | Mature, adult oriented | Cautious |
| Careful | Businesslike | Expensive |
| Organized | Clean | Upscale |
| Innovative | Consistent | Cheap |
| Knowledgeable | Experienced | Organized |
| Modern | Stable | Simple |
| Professional | Competent | Specialized |
| Trustworthy | Concerned | General |
| Understanding | Confused | Flexible |
| Attention to fine detail | Glasses oriented | Structured |
| Conservative | Patient centered | Rural |
| Daring | Slow | Urban |
| Original | Inefficient | Blue collar |
| Nostalgic | Efficient | White collar |
| Wide selection | Friendly | |

Comments:

This is your identity—if it's real. A way of ascertaining if it is real is by asking friends or patients to complete the exercise for your office. Does their response match your perceptions?

# Reasons Patients Leave Your Practice

If your records are arranged so that you can do this easily, pull cards on 100 patients you've not seen in the past year. Have a staff member call and suggest scheduling a follow-up exam or care. If they're reluctant or won't commit, try probing for reasons. Tally what you can, using the following list. Computer programs may facilitate this. Also, patient surveys that have been returned may give you the necessary feedback.

| Reason | Number of Patients |
|---|---|
| No longer reachable at residence phone | |
| No longer reachable at job phone | |
| Relocated away from local area | |
| Deceased | |
| Resident of long-term or assisted living facility | |
| Uses different vision coverage | |
| Uses closed panel HMO for vision | |
| Personality conflict with ECP | |
| Personality conflict with staff member | |
| Inconvenient office hours | |
| Excessive waiting time for an appointment | |
| Excessive waiting time during prior exams | |
| Excessive fees | |
| Not satisfied with prior products received | |
| Not satisfied with prior services received | |
| Quality of prior experience was less than expected | |
| Other (specify) | |

Modified from Building. AOA Practice Enhancement Program I. St. Louis, MO: American Optometric Association; 1984.

# Marketing During the Patient Visit

| Marketing Technique | Using Success-fully | Using but Needs Im-provement | Not Using and Don't Want To | Not Appro-priate |
|---|---|---|---|---|
| **Before patient enters office** | | | | |
| Phone hold message | | | | |
| Smiles | | | | |
| Welcome to the office | | | | |
| Office brochure | | | | |
| Biographical sketch | | | | |
| Information packets | | | | |
| Practice location | | | | |
| Building appearance | | | | |
| Parking lot | | | | |
| Window displays | | | | |
| **In the reception area** | | | | |
| Office appearance | | | | |
| Reception area design | | | | |
| Color | | | | |
| Décor | | | | |
| Furniture | | | | |
| Staff greeting | | | | |
| Staff appearance | | | | |
| Attire | | | | |
| Attitude | | | | |
| Attention | | | | |
| Library | | | | |
| Electronic bulletin board | | | | |

| Marketing Technique | Using Success-fully | Using but Needs Im-provement | Not Using and Don't Want To | Not Appro-priate |
|---|---|---|---|---|
| Videos | | | | |
| Counter cards | | | | |
| Product brochures | | | | |
| Samples | | | | |
| Demonstrators | | | | |
| Business cards | | | | |
| Ad and publicity reprints | | | | |
| Refreshments | | | | |
| Treats | | | | |
| Television | | | | |
| Reading materials | | | | |
| Miscellaneous | | | | |
| Bathrooms | | | | |
| Music | | | | |
| **During patient's history and pretesting** | | | | |
| History form | | | | |
| History questions | | | | |
| Posters | | | | |
| Testimonials | | | | |
| Diplomas, awards | | | | |
| News articles | | | | |
| Photos of celebrity patients | | | | |
| Equipment | | | | |
| Explanations of benefits | | | | |
| Scripts for assistant | | | | |
| Dispensing mats, etc. | | | | |
| **During the exam** | | | | |
| Exam room | | | | |
| Neatness | | | | |
| Saying hello | | | | |

| Marketing Technique | Using Success-fully | Using but Needs Im-provement | Not Using and Don't Want To | Not Appro-priate |
|---|---|---|---|---|
| Explaining test procedures | | | | |
| Models | | | | |
| Pictures | | | | |
| Lenses | | | | |
| Written materials | | | | |
| Articles | | | | |
| Books | | | | |
| Samples | | | | |
| Saying goodbye | | | | |
| Referral cards | | | | |
| Exam summaries | | | | |
| **In the dispensary** | | | | |
| Décor | | | | |
| Sales training | | | | |
| Lens packages | | | | |
| Frame displays | | | | |
| Merchandise displays | | | | |
| Gift packages | | | | |
| Free slips and receipts | | | | |
| **After the visit** | | | | |
| Follow-up | | | | |
| Phone calls | | | | |
| Cards and letters | | | | |
| Stationery | | | | |
| Newsletters | | | | |
| Special invitations | | | | |
| Gifts | | | | |
| Recall | | | | |

## Notes

1. Relationship marketing grows long-term success. *Modern Money.* 1998;2(1):1–4.
2. Data taken from CDA Weisenberger, Thomson Financial, Rockville, MD, 2000.
3. Greiner D, Kinni T. *1001 Ways to Keep Customers Coming Back.* Rocklin, CA: Prima Publishing; 1999:139.
4. W. D. Sullins, Jr., e-mail, Survey of successful marketing tactics, July 29, 2000.
5. Cziepel J, Congram C, Shanahan J. Exploring the concept of loyalty in services. In: *The Service Challenge: Integrating for Competitive Advantage.* Chicago: American Marketing Association; 1987:91–94.
6. Solomon MR, Suprenant C, Czepiel JA, et al. A role theory perspective on dyadic interactions: The service encounter. *Journal of Marketing.* March 1985:99–111.
7. Public opinion on health care issues. *American Medical News.* October 13, 1997;30(38):12.
8. Peltier J, Boyt T, Schibrowsky J. Relationship building. *Marketing Health Services.* Fall 1998:17–24.
9. Berry L, Parasuraman A. *Marketing Services.* New York: Free Press; 1991.
10. Christopher M, Payne A, Ballantyne D. *Relationship Marketing.* Oxford: Butterworth–Heinemann; 1996.
11. J. Mallinger, e-mail, Survey of successful marketing tactics, August 3, 2000.
12. M. Silverman, e-mail, Survey of successful marketing tactics, July 25, 2000.
13. Leenders M, Blenkhorn D. *Reverse Marketing: The New Buyer-Supplier Relationship.* New York: Free Press; 1988:8.
14. Masson R. User vendor relationships. *International Journal of Quality and Reliability Management.* 1985;3(2):31–37.
15. M. Spitzer, e-mail, Survey of successful marketing tactics, July 25, 2000.
16. D. Howard, e-mail, Survey of successful marketing tactics, July 25, 2000.
17. Maister D. *Professional Service Firm Management.* Boston: Maister Associates; 1989:78.

18. Gummesson E. The new marketing: Developing long term interactive relationships. *Long Range Planning.* 1987;20(4):10–20.
19. Treacy M, Wiersema F. *The Discipline of Market Leaders: Choose Your Customers, Narrow Your Focus, and Dominate Your Market.* Reading, MA: Addison-Wesley; 1997.
20. LaLonde B, Zinszer P. *Customer Service: Meaning and Measurement.* Chicago: NCPDM; 1976.
21. Walton D. Branding your practice. *Dental Practice and Finance.* November–December 1997:25–26.
22. Petromilli M, Michalczyk D. Your most valuable asset. *Marketing Health Services.* Summer 1999:5–9.
23. Shea W. The patient partner paradigm. *Managed Healthcare News.* March 1998:33.
24. Osler R. The name game: tips on how to get it right. *Marketing News.* September, 14, 1998;32(19):50.
25. Berry L, Lefkowith E, Clark T. In services, what's in a name? *Harvard Business Review.* September–October 1988:28–30.
26. McCarthy R. What price brand identity? *Managed Healthcare News.* November 1997;13(11):14.
27. Levinson JC. *Guerilla Marketing Attack.* Boston: Houghton Mifflin; 1989.
28. Hayes J. As long as it's free. *Forbes.* January 30, 1995;155:72–73.
29. Robertson K. Strategically desirable brand name characteristics. *Journal of Consumer Marketing.* Fall 1989;6:61–71.
30. Dolliver M. Ad showcase. *Adweek's Marketing Week.* August 20, 1990:31–32.
31. Henderson P, Cote J. Guidelines for selecting and modifying logos. *Journal of Marketing.* April 1998;62:14–30.
32. Joseph S. *Marketing the Physician Practice.* Chicago: American Marketing Association; 2000:64.
33. Baker S. Improving service and increasing patient satisfaction. *Family Practice Management.* July–August 1998:29–33.
34. Schneider B, Bowen D. *Winning the Service Game.* Boston: Harvard Business School Press; 1995:233.
35. Woodcock E. The telephone: Managing demand. *Medical Practice Management.* July–August 1999:19–22.
36. LeBoeuf M. *How to Win Customers and Keep Them for Life.* San Francisco: The Berkley Publishing Group; 1989.

# CHAPTER 6

# Managing the Marketing Mix

## Value Chain Concept

The contemporary value chain concept in eyecare has its foundation in the principles described by Michael Porter in *Competitive Advantage*, his classic text on business strategy.[1] The value chain consists of the systems and operations that a practice uses to deliver premium value to its customers. The goal is to offer a level of performance that ultimately translates into superior revenues and profit. The value chain process starts when the ECP acquires the resources necessary to deliver what is promised (inbound logistics). Next, the ECP develops specific "operations" (practice work processes) that will deliver the products and services to patients (outbound logistics) in a cost-saving manner.[1] These two steps are combined with the marketing and sales function to make potential patients aware of the superior value the practice offers. The final result is a patient perception that focuses on high-quality service to "keep them happy." The value in this model is either the worth of the services patients purchase or the price they are willing to pay for what they receive.[1] The implication for eyecare is that, to earn patient loyalty, the ECP must provide value above and beyond what patients expect. This chapter demonstrates how the marketing function enhances the value chain within the eyecare setting and introduces the basic tools available to assist the ECP in marketing endeavors.

## Components of the Marketing Mix, the Four *P*s Model

The term *marketing mix* describes the important functions and components that compose the overall marketing program. "The marketing mix refers to the apportionment of effort—the combination, the designing, and the integration of the various elements of marketing—into a program that, on the basis of an appraisal of the market forces, will best achieve the objectives of an enterprise at a given time."[2] The concept originated in the 1960s with the work of N. H. Borden, at the Harvard Business School, who suggested 12 elements be considered when developing a marketing plan, as shown in Table 6–1.[3] Since its introduction, the wide acceptance of the marketing mix is due to its simplification into four parts by Professor Jerome McCarthy, known as the *four P*s:

1. *Price*. Fees charged patients and terms of sales.
2. *Product*. Services and products the practice offers.
3. *Place*. Physical distribution that makes products and services available to patients.
4. *Promotion*. All communication activities the practice performs.

**Table 6–1   Components of a Marketing Program**

| |
| --- |
| Product planning |
| Pricing |
| Branding |
| Channels of distribution |
| Personal selling |
| Advertising |
| Promotions |
| Packaging |
| Display |
| Servicing |
| Physical handling |
| Fact finding and analysis |

Reprinted with permission from Borden N. The concept of the marketing mix. In: Schwartz G, ed. *Science in Marketing*. New York: John Wiley; 1965:386–397.

An acronym that evolved from the "four *Ps*" is AIDAS, which describes the desired sequence of actions a marketer must perform to achieve satisfied customers:[4]

*Attention.* Gain the patient's attention.
*Interest.* The patient develops interest.
*Desire.* The patient desires to pursue the purchase.
*Action.* The patient acts on the desire.
*Satisfaction.* The patient is satisfied with the outcome.

**Limitations of the Four *P* Model**

Since the 1960s, the classic four *P* model has been used by marketers to develop the specific marketing mix or tactics that make up the overall marketing strategy.[5] However, the model has certain restrictions due to its simplistic approach, "which has resulted in a lack of empirical study into the key marketing variables, how they are perceived and used by marketing managers and a neglect of process in favour of structure."[6] These limitations can be overcome by expanding the model to include two additional *P*s:

*People.*[7] Consideration of employees and training as a vital resource for practice success.
*Performance.*[8] Satisfying patient's needs and wants through customer service.

Patient needs or desires affect the different components of the marketing mix (four *P*s) that an ECP uses to develop overall marketing strategy. Patient attitudes or lifestyle usage patterns affect the types of *products* ECPs decide to offer. A noticeable number of patients requesting information on a specific product may signal the need to offer that product or at least information about the product's use and its advantages. Patient attitudes and local area demographics influence the *promotion* component of the marketing mix. Informing patients about what the practice offers and designing marketing messages to appeal to potential patients will vary with the perception of patient interest in the practice's products or services. A patient's eagerness to research comparative price levels and develop a reasonable budget to spend on specific products or services directly affects the *price* component of the marketing mix. The patient's ease in reaching your office influences the *place* component of the marketing mix, specifically your accessibility, your hours of operation, and the methods you select for patients to receive your products and services. Recognizing and rewarding the input from the *people* that you employ to get and keep patients in your practice will enhance overall performance. Finally, practice *performance* should lead to patient satisfaction as the outcome of reliable and timely operations.

Controlling and managing the variables affecting decision making in traditional areas of price policy, product and service offering, and promotional activities will reinforce your ability to achieve your desired goals and satisfy your consumers. Pricing takes into account costs, desired profit, and sensitivity to competitive forces that affect your practice's profitability. Product and service offerings include an array of existing and new products and services that patients receive in your office.

Many of the tactics used by ECPs place emphasis on promotion as the primary marketing mix function. Promotional activities include all personal and nonpersonal selling, advertising, public relations, and other media communications used to reach your target market. The prices an ECP charges can be used to differentiate a practice, but most often, fees are predetermined by third parties or usual and customary in a given area. The place function includes both internal and external methods used to deliver products, services, and marketing messages and often is included within the promotion function. The product to concentrate on delivering will be the topic of discussion in the next chapter, covering patient satisfaction and service quality.

## When Service Is the Product

In addition to the typical tangible products (spectacles and contact lenses) consumers purchase in an ECP's office, examination and dispensing also belong in the category of service-product. According to the American Marketing Association, the service-product is composed of these characteristics:[9]

1. Substantially intangible.
2. Exchanged directly from producer to user.
3. Cannot be transported or stored.
4. Difficult to identify, its existence coincides with its consumption.
5. Comprises inseparable tangible elements.
6. Includes important customer involvement.
7. Ownership or title cannot be sold.

An understanding of the unusual requirements inherent in the marketing of services enhances the success of any marketing program you endeavor to undertake. This includes the intangible quality of services, which does not allow you to appeal to a patient's senses or separate the service from you. It is impossible to standardize service, since nearly all encounters can be considered unique. The demand for services typically fluctuates, requiring the efficient utilization of resources during lower demand periods and the ability to accommodate excess demand in peak periods. Finally, services marketing demands greater creativity. Table 6–2 identifies six critical differences between products and services as influential factors in an ECP's marketing decisions.

**An ECP has several opportunities during the patient encounter to offer extraordinary service.** These involve the physical setting, including the sights, sounds, and odors the patient experiences. Interpersonal interactions you and your staff have with patients, such as willingness to accommodate, can influence a patient's perception of the visit. Other areas to look for adding value are the speed and cost of service or moments where you can interject unexpected enhancements. Ask yourself, Ultimately, what do I strive to achieve in my practice? If the answer is patient satisfaction through offering high-quality service, then a moment of truth analysis can confirm if you are accomplishing your goal.

Of paramount importance for the ECP is to design a service delivery system that achieves the highest possible perceived quality by the greatest number of patients. One technique the ECP can use to detect, prevent, and remediate service encounter weaknesses is a detailed schematic flow chart of each step of your practice's service processes, called *service blueprinting*. This is

**Table 6–2   The Difference Between Products and Services**

1. *Product.* The patient owns a tangible object.
   *Service.* The patient owns an intangible memory that can't be sold or passed on.
2. *Product.* The goal of producing a product is uniformity for all units.
   *Service.* The delivery goal is unique, each patient experience is special.
3. *Product.* Samples can be inventoried and previewed.
   *Service.* Occurs at the moment, no stockpiling.
4. *Product.* The patient is the end user, not involved in production process.
   *Service.* The patient is a participant and full partner in creating the service.
5. *Product.* Quality control compares final output to predetermined specifications.
   *Service.* The patient assesses quality by comparing expectations to experience.
6. *Product.* Improper examples can be withdrawn or replaced.
   *Service.* Inadequate performance results in apologies or refunds or both.

Adapted from Zemke R. The emerging art of service management. *Training.* January 1992: 36–42.

accomplished through diagraming the patient visit cycle using a flowchart to develop both a plan and diagnostic report, in turn adding shape and visual recognition to the components of the intangible service encounter in your office.[10]

The two key components of service blueprints are lines of visibility and fail points. Procedures not visible to the patient are considered behind the line, while those the patient directly experiences or observes are above the line.[10] It is important to remember that service processes patients experience often are the result of backroom work and this area should not be overlooked when developing or modifying practice operations. Fail points are the processes most likely to breakdown or exhibit failure. Identifying fail points is closely associated with but not the same thing as moment of truth analysis. Identifying fail points directs attention to the need for special or additional training, tighter controls or inspection to detail, and adding additional steps to or redesigning parts of the service delivery process. Minimizing the probability of failure, breakdown, or patient misperception should be a primary objective when designing the practice's operational processes.

Several tactics are available for the ECP to continually monitor, assess, and refine the practice's operational effectiveness. Employing "disguised" patients to help you assess the performance of your staff can be enlightening but produces occasional discord. The comments made by a professional shopper hired to evaluate office staff and its patient interaction can be considered intrusive by staff members. Any suggestions for remediation should be made objectively, based on unwanted behavior not on personality. Patients can be sent surveys periodically to collect feedback. Finally, you can seek staff input about patient comments, giving special attention to the analysis and cause of patient complaints.

## Determining a Marketing Budget

The actual amount of money you allocate for marketing depends on your business objectives. Whatever the amount, the commitment should be for a reasonable period of time and justified. An ECP with an attitude that mimics "we'll spend as little money as we have to on marketing, see how it works, and then decide whether or not to continue" reflects a practice that may be marketing out of desperation as opposed to reaching a predetermined goal. The concept of the zero-based marketing budget requires that, before any money is allocated, anyone responsible for spending marketing dollars must justify the need and demonstrate how the money will be spent. Money spent on marketing should be considered an investment in the future of the practice. At a minimum, you can consider the intangible benefits of marketing or return on your investment as staying in business, staying ahead of the competition, attracting new patients, and retaining former ones.

Your budget should not place too much emphasis on any one particular product, activity, or channel; rather, it should be part of a program where one marketing tactic feeds off others to augment the power and overall effectiveness. Any program you develop should include[11]

1. Self-promotion through point-of-purchase material. This could be a copy of a newspaper article about something you did or an award plaque on the wall of the waiting room.
2. Media relations using educational and informative messages, including newsletters and in-office brochures.
3. Advertising in mass media channels such as the Yellow Pages and local newspapers.

Most budgetary decisions that relate to advertising and promotion are aimed at attracting new customers to the business as the primary objective. The range of expenditure for this purpose as a percent of gross revenue varies anywhere from 2% for industrial product companies to 10% for businesses that focus on consumer products.[11] It would be justified in most established ECP settings to allocate 4–6% of revenues for promotions. For either startup locations or the introduction of new services to existing locations, an additional 2–6% would not be unreasonable to achieve patient awareness and gain market share.

Several different methods can be used when determining the amount of funds a business should allocate for marketing, as shown in Table 6–3. The first method is to simply use an arbitrarily chosen, previously used percentage that is applied to the past year's gross revenue. This figure does not consider any special

**Table 6–3    Methods to Determine a Marketing Budget**

1. Previously used percentage of revenue.
2. Spend what you can afford.
3. Reactive, spur of the moment, not planned.
4. Competitive parity.
5. Amount required to achieve predetermined objectives.
6. Amount based on estimated cost of acquiring and retaining a new patient and number of new patients desired.

Modified from Krueger J. Developing a marketing budget. *Target Marketing*. October 1996; 19(10):118–120.

communication programs or opportunities that sporadically occur in your local market as new product offerings or one-time sales.

The second method comes from a spend-what-you-can-afford mindset. This method often results in inadequate funding due to the conservative nature of the decision and evolves from the fear of squandering hard-earned dollars, often the case in a downturn economy. However, it is important to allocate a greater amount to marketing during these slower periods to entice patients to make appointments.

The third method takes a reactive position, more from desperation than planning. The position often is characterized by procrastination or a decision maker who avoids establishing a more formal approach to marketing. This may be due to the belief in a false negative stigma associated with marketing by health care professionals, a commonly held belief prior to the 1980s.

The fourth method is led by marketplace dynamics, keeping pace with the competition. Competitive parity requires the ECP to monitor, through competitor intelligence, the level of competitive spending and match it. However, should the matching amount be based on actual dollar outlay or percentage of gross revenue? Through a diligent monitoring program, you determine your competition is spending 5% of its gross revenue on media marketing. If you decide to match the amount, unless your gross revenues are the same as your competitor, the amount you each spend still will be different.

A fifth method requires the ECP to determine a desired future revenue goal from a specific marketing program and make allocations based on the projected cost of the required marketing to achieve that goal. From previous experience, you know that you realize a $5,000 gross revenue increase through a mail coupon offer that costs $1,000. Next year, if you want to increase your revenue by $20,000, you would allocate $4,000 for coupon mailings.

The final method takes into account the lifetime value of a patient, as previously discussed. The ECP decides an allowable cost to acquire each new patient and retain those patients over a planned time frame in different categories, such as contact lens or refractive surgery. Decide how many new patients in each category your practice can satisfy with the level of service required.

Multiply that number of patients by the projected cost to acquire a patient, then allocate funds to each category. Simply put: "determine how much you're willing to pay for a customer, then determine how many you want in the coming year . . . and multiply."[12] DiMark Marketing, a specialty database marketing firm in Pennsylvania, believes the cost of acquiring a new Medicare patient ranges from $200 to $1,000 per member depending on the tactics used.[13] With proper analysis, the ECP will be able to determine ahead of time what marketing effort will be required to produce the desired results.

The ECP should answer several questions to ensure that allocated marketing funds will be spent wisely.[14]

1. Can you link every dollar you plan to spend to defined practice goals, or is some of the money allocated for marketing tactics you always rely on?
2. Have you distributed the total marketing budget in a way that reflects the relative importance of specific programs? Don't spend an excessively large portion of your total budget on any one product or service unless you anticipate enough income can be generated from that specific product or service. Exceptions to this might be new products that you believe have great profit potential or aggressive competitors who attempt to capture market share and threaten your present patient base.
3. Do the patient groups and products that offer the highest profit potential receive the most dollars? Don't allocate half your total budget to a program targeted at a product or patient segment that, at best, can contribute only a 5% increase in new revenues.
4. Are you using the proper marketing mix and combination of channels without diluting the impact of your message? Having your practice identity circulated in every part of your practice's drawing area in all possible media formats is very impressive, but is it at the expense of not making a lasting impression on a significant number of potential patients?
5. Monitoring and tracking the results of your marketing program is the final task you should perform to assess the effec-

tiveness of specific tactics in reaching your objectives. Can you determine your cost in acquiring a new patient and what the lifetime worth of that patient is to your practice? Do you know how effective your marketing is in preventing patients from leaving your office? Is the amount allocated for marketing appropriate to the size of your business, the goals you wish to achieve, and the amount your competitors are spending? Ideally, you would like to optimize the effectiveness of every marketing dollar you spend. Pennsylvania department store entrepreneur John Wanamaker said, "Half my advertising is wasted; I just don't know which half."[11] Refer to Table 6–4 for century-old wisdom on advertising.

## Personal Selling

Probably the best opportunity the ECP has to influence patient decision making is during the case summary at the end of a patient exam. Coincidentally, this happens to be the least expensive marketing tactic available to you. A study performed by Genesis Training Solutions concludes that your presentation should be organized, informal, relaxed, and conversational in style.[15] Avoid taking a hard-sell approach; rather, be informative and educational while suggesting specific products the patient should use. A technique used by Dr. Denise Howard of Bloomington, Indiana, is

> spend the extra 2–3 minutes that it takes to ask about the grandchildren, the new job, or the trip to Europe. My assistants gather as much information as possible and that gives me more time to educate my patients and answer their questions. We also never try to sell a patient a service or product that will not benefit them but we do take the time to inform our patients about new developments.[16]

Clarify the tangible and intangible benefits the patient receives by following your recommendations and justify the cost with qualitative cost-benefit support. Always use facts to add support and make your goal for the patient believable. If the patient is unsure or states, "I have been happy using _____ [a specific brand of spectacle contact lens]. Why should I change to

**Table 6–4   How Often Should You Advertise?**

The answer may surprise you. What are people actually thinking about as they read your ad in a local paper? Thomas Smith, a 19th-century London businessman, offered the following advice to advertisers in 1885. It is still applicable today.

1. The first time people look at any given ad, they don't even see it.
2. The second time, they don't notice it.
3. The third time, they are aware that it is there.
4. The fourth time, they have a fleeting sense that they've seen it somewhere before.
5. The fifth time, they actually read the ad.
6. The sixth time, they thumb their nose at it.
7. The seventh time, they start to get a little irritated with it.
8. The eighth time, they start to think, "Here's that confounded ad again."
9. The ninth time, they start to wonder if they may be missing out on something.
10. The tenth time, they ask their friends and neighbors if they've tried it.
11. The eleventh time, they wonder how the company is paying for all these ads.
12. The twelfth time, they start to think that it must be a good product.
13. The thirteenth time, they start to feel the product has value.
14. The fourteenth time, they start to remember wanting a product exactly like this for a long time.
15. The fifteenth time, they start to yearn for it because they can't afford to buy it.
16. The sixteenth time, they accept the fact that they will buy it sometime in the future.
17. The seventeenth time, they make a note to buy the product.
18. The eighteenth time, they curse their poverty for not allowing them to buy this terrific product.
19. The nineteenth time, they count their money very carefully.
20. The twentieth time prospects see the ad, they buy what it is offering.

In other words, if your ad campaigns aren't showing a return after six weeks, don't give up hope.

Reprinted with permission from The Winning Edge, Sales and Marketing Report 2000. Chicago: Lawrence Ragan Communications, Inc., 2000.

what you recommend?" Agree with the patient that his or her present brand is a good product, but point out the advantages the new brand of product offers over their present brand. Use a persuasive argument to explain why the outcome will be favorable for the patient, show confidence, and be prepared to answer any what-if or negative questions.

Another unique opportunity to increase patient referrals can be the result of a personal relationship you develop with bridal salon owners.[17] Ask the owner if you can put display posters promoting the advantages of wearing clear or colored contact lenses rather than glasses to enhance the appearance of the bride and groom in their wedding photos. For every referral you receive, credit the bridal owner's personal account with your office. Figure 6–1 shows a sample letter to send to a bridal salon owner.

---

XYZ Wedding Days
123 Any Street
Anywhere, USA

Dear Mr. Weddingbells,

As a way to enhance both of our businesses, I would like to suggest a referral arrangement from which we would both benefit. As a prominent eye-care provider in our community, I offer a service that would be well received and valued by your customers. My practice is capable of improving the appearance of brides on their wedding day through the use of contact lenses to replace eyeglasses or colored contact lenses to enhance their eye color.

What I would want from you are referrals of brides and grooms to my office for contact lens fittings. In exchange for these referrals, I would establish a personal account for you or your family members and credit your account $50 for each referral to be used toward the purchase of eyewear. At your convenience, please call my office and I will be happy to give you a personal tour, and if such an arrangement seems advantageous to you, I invite you to be my guest for lunch to discuss the details further.

Respectfully,


Peter Eyesight, O.D.

---

**Figure 6–1    Sample letter to establish relationship with bridal salon.**

## Cross Selling

Have you ever wondered why a patient may use your practice for only a portion of their eyecare needs and purchase additional products or services from another office. One reason for the patient to go elsewhere is that your practice does not offer what he or she wants. This can be simply rectified at your discretion by expanding your inventory. A more fundamental reason for a patient going elsewhere is a lack of knowledge about all that your practice provides. This can be resolved through a well-developed cross-selling program, performed in an informative manner from a patient education approach not a hard-sell tactic. It seems that an ECP must constantly remind patients of all the products and services that are available from their office, especially for recently released products or newly acquired services.

If revenue enhancement is one of the ECP's goals, it is much easier to achieve this by marketing additional services and products to existing patients than it is to increase your patient base by marketing to new patients. The ECP has several opportunities to cross-sell directly to patients including:[18]

1. Direct mail or e-mail.
2. In-office signs.
3. Patient lounge videos and computers.
4. Open house.
5. On-hold telephone message.

Direct mail announcements can be incorporated into regularly mailed newsletters or individual-targeted mailings for specific patient groups. Either of these can be potentially supported by co-op funds from suppliers. E-mail will appeal to your more high-tech oriented patients, but requires the ECP to maintain a database of e-mail addresses. In-office posters and signs can often be obtained at no cost from manufacturers or distributors and should be displayed in the patient lounge or other prominent, visible spot that attracts patient attention. The patient lounge can also be used for multimedia and educational video presentations. A computer can be programmed to allow patients to work through various menus about ophthalmic conditions and associated products and services. An open house offers the opportunity to showcase new products but also makes patients aware of other products your practice offers. On-hold messages are becoming more prevalent in all health care providers' practices. These messages can suggest prevention and remediation of ocular conditions they may have as well as new products and services. Take care that the message does not leave the patient on hold too long or else they may become frustrated, hang up, and seek another practice.

## Print Media

### Direct Mail

Direct mail is one of the more commonly used mechanisms to reach patients with targeted marketing messages. Many different items are included in this category: recall notices, newsletters, sale and new product announcements, new associates and alliances, eyecare insurance, and wellness information. To prevent wasted dollars on printing and postage, a few rules apply to insure higher response rates from your mailings.

1. Send information that is relevant to the receiver. You will probably have a less than optimal response if you send material about new PALs or low vision to a family in their twenties with a young child.
2. Target and choose the most likely audience to care about and appreciate the benefits you are offering.
3. Use an updated address list. A larger than expected returned mail rate may signal your mailing list and addresses are out of date.
4. If you are going to do a bulk mailing, you should pick 100 names randomly and do a trial run. This gives you the opportunity to assess the response to the offer and make any changes you believe necessary to improve the response for the full mailing.
5. Use individual, personalized headings in the address and salutation whenever possible. This may require an investment into

specialized management software but should eliminate many recipients from throwing away the letter before they open it.

6. Use "buzz" words that attract attention: "free trial," "guarantee," and "prevention" are all applicable.
7. Monitor your response rate to know what works and what did not for your next mailing.

Whenever you mail an office introduction brochure, keep in mind that less is more. The content should be concise and easy to read, using easily identified headings, bullets, and numbered lists for emphasis. Make sure you enclose a personalized, signed cover letter, not a photocopy or preprinted "Dear patient" form letter. If an appointment already has been made, refer the patient to your practice website and add a patient history form to be completed and a self-addressed stamped envelope. Put the information in your database and use the opportunity to offer enhanced service by informing the patient of what to expect on the first visit and what unique or special service and products your practice offers. The actual brochure, at a minimum, should include the information listed in Table 6–5. Direct mail was successful for Stephen Sokol, O.D., of La Mirada, California. He states that

> my practice is 29 years old. I worked for a gentleman for three years before that in a discount store. When the store closed, I moved one mile north—joined the La Mirada Chamber of Commerce and put out a mass letter to all citizenry in La Mirada, with my picture on the letter stating

**Table 6–5    Information for Practice Brochure**

Brief bio of the ECP: education, professional highlights, and principal clinical interests.

Staff members: List positions and training.

Directions, map, hours of operation, and website address.

Emergency contacts.

Practice mission and intent (see Chapter 2).

Plans accepted and payment policies.

Specialized patient services.

Infection control procedures.

Website address.

that this is Dr. Stephen P. Sokol, formerly with Dr. _____, and never had a starvation period.[19]

A universally used, but frequently overlooked, marketing tactic is the professional business and appointment card. Is your business card the traditional 3.5" × 2" white rectangle or is it an innovative shape with a uniquely identifying logo?[20] You can have both a business card for marketing and a separate appointment card as a reminder; they need not be the same, because they serve different purposes. Does your card enhance your image? Convey a desire to motivate an inquiry? Offer ideas about your practice? Include your website and e-mail address? If you consider your business card another channel for delivering your marketing message, would it be different than the one you presently have? If so, you might want to revamp your card.

## Yellow Pages

Long considered the most commonly used method of advertising, Yellow Pages advertising has become quite expensive and less profitable in the past decade, especially in urban areas, due to managed care. However, the opposite can be said about certain suburban and rural locations. Managed care, for many ECPs, has turned mass media into a medium that offers a less than desirable profit. In other areas, especially less densely populated suburban and rural areas, Yellow Pages advertising still is essential for attracting new patients. You can determine how successful Yellow Pages advertising is in attracting new patients by obtaining a "call accounting service" that measures volume and compiles statistics based on caller identification from the phone company. Yellow Pages advertising should primarily and visually emphasize the services you offer by addressing the message to potential patients unfamiliar with your practice.

Research studies based on consumer eye movements while viewing the Yellow Pages offer the following suggestions to gain a higher consumer response to Yellow Pages advertising:[21]

1. Large display ads were observed 93% of the time but plain ads only 26%.

2. Ads with color were observed before and 21% longer than ads without color.
3. 96% of the ads with graphics were viewed, but graphics did not gain initial consumer attention while color did.
4. The larger the ad, the better chance it is noticed, and the position that the ad occupies on the page has a large influence.
5. The majority of consumers scan a page alphabetically; the earlier in the alphabet your business name appears on the page, the better positioned to be observed.
6. Ads with low amounts of information were viewed less than those with high amounts, but ads appearing crowded with too much information were viewed less.

The Yellow Pages Publishing Association found that 31% of consumers undecided on a health care provider were influenced by what they saw in the Yellow Pages.[22] If you should decide to use Yellow Pages advertising, Table 6–6 shows a few suggestions. Appendix 6–2 lists numerous additional marketing tactics ECPs may use to promote their practices. Yellow Pages often are used by both price shoppers and as a last resort for finding an ECP. Because of this, the no-show rate is higher than from other referral sources. One source reported a 49% no-show rate with Yellow Pages compared to 26% overall for the practice.[23]

**Table 6–6   Yellow Pages Advertising**

1. Include information on specialty services that set you apart from other ECPs.
2. Place your ad in phone books that go only to your location's drawing area.
3. Describe consumer services you offer, such as credit cards accepted, insurance accepted and claims filled out, extended hours.
4. List in more than one category.
5. Listings are in alphabetical order, if you want to be first, change your practice name to one that starts with *A*.
6. Monitor and track results to determine worthiness and return on investment.

Adapted from Wilkins K, Borglum K. Letting your fingers do the walking pays off. *Practice Marketing and Management*. May 1998:61.

## Push-Pull Strategy

A popular marketing tactic deserving a brief explanation is the push-pull strategy.[2] Push strategy occurs when manufacturers and vendors offer incentives to intermediaries, in this case ECPs, to offer and promote their product to patients. Incentives could include volume discount, point-of-purchase promotion materials or funds, and in-office staff training. Pull strategy occurs when manufacturers and vendors create demand at the consumer level by reaching patients through advertising or direct mail as the primary target for their promotional efforts. The goal is to have patients go into the ECP office and ask for a specific product and brand. An example of this is when contact lens manufacturers use magazine media to promote their specialty brand of lens resulting in patients requesting these during their exams.

## Setting Fees

The price an ECP chooses for products and services can be determined by comparison with other ECPs and the going rate in the local area. This information should not be obtained through a formal survey as part of a provider network or the ECP could be in violation of the Sherman Anti-Trust Law, being considered a form of price-fixing.[24] This does not take into account the direct costs involved in delivering the product or service nor the desired profit per unit delivered.

Another technique used to set fees considers the relative worth of each product or service an ECP delivers as a function of a third party's predetermined fee schedules. These typically are low, and when ECPs choose to devalue their services by using low prices, the danger exists that the patient will perceive the services as not being valuable, questioning either the ECP's expertise or effort in the delivery of such services. On the flip side are excessively high fees. If not justified, these can prevent patients from making the first appointment. Appendix 6–1 offers a checklist that may help when setting or changing the practice fee structure.

The price of goods and services often is the first point of resistance a patient will comment about.

> Price is the only element of the marketing mix that generates revenue; all other elements incur cost. However, price is important for another reason customers use price as a clue about the product. Price can build up the customer's confidence in the product—or lessen it. Price can raise customer expectations ("this is expensive, it had better be good") or lower them ("you get what you pay for").[25]

A price that is extremely high may be perceived by patients as a "rip-off or not good value." A high price may require added support and justification through patient education as to the value of the product.

Value is the total benefit received for the total cost incurred, price being only one component of total cost. Speed, courtesy, and reassurance are examples of additional factors in the value patients perceive. Your price offers patients insight into the quality of your service and products. Carefully choose the level to position the products and services to be offered. Will you offer basic no frills, economical, value-oriented products and services or premium class with all the add-ons?

Setting the "right price" indicates concern for the patient's welfare and offers a clear strategy on positioning your services in the marketplace. Table 6–7 identifies different ways to use price in combination with the volume of service offered. In one strategy, referred to as *skimming*,[26] initially the ECP sets a high price for a product or service and focuses all marketing efforts at patient groups most willing to pay the high fee. Slowly, prices are lowered to capture a greater volume of patients who are only willing to spend less. The opposite of this fee strategy is *penetration*, where the ECP starts at a low fee to gain a larger portion of the potential market share and abruptly preempts competitors. The downside of this strategy is the loss of higher profits, especially from those patients who would be willing to pay more.[8] Eventually, prices could rise as demand increases or features are added to the product, resulting in increased profit. A follow-the-leader price strategy uses a specific competitor against which the ECP sets fees. A possible disadvantage of this strategy is retaliation by the competitor, resulting in a downward spiral on prices. A variable price strategy uses more than one fee for the services and products to give concessions to certain patients. Caution

**Table 6–7   Price as a Differentiation Strategy**

More service for more cost than the competition.

More service for the same cost as the competition.

More service for less cost than the competition.

The same amount of service for less cost than the competition.

Less service for less cost than the competition.

Adapted from Kotler P. *Kotler on Marketing*. New York: Free Press; 1999.

must be used if the ECP applies this strategy to ensure that compliance with federal regulations is maintained and the policy does not prove to be discriminatory.

## Tracking the Effectiveness of Promotional Tactics

A decision often is required to determine which tactics to use to market the services of a particular office. It would be very worthwhile to know how effective the options are when compared to each other or which option yields the best return for the costs incurred. A simple table, properly constructed, can reveal valuable information comparing the cost and benefits of any marketing tactic you have used in the past.[27] With the insight gained from tracking previous results, you are better informed, and thus more secure, in your choice of future tactics. An example of a cost-benefit marketing tactic monitoring table is shown in Table 6–8.

For this example, a trial marketing program is considered, using a 3-month period in which five different tactics are selected. These are the column headings of Table 6–8, each identified by a letter, A through E. The Explanation of Marketing Tactics Cost gives a brief explanation of the various tactics, and associated costs. The first row of Table 6–8 shows the cost of each marketing tactic used. Subsequent rows list the quantifiable results from each of the tactics. The values are derived by tracking and compiling the response from each program, recording the number of patient inquiries, patient exams, products dispensed, and resulting gross revenue.

**Table 6–8    Cost-Benefit Marketing Monitor Chart, Showing Various Quarterly Revenue Sources for a Trial Marketing Program**

|  | A. Yellow Pages | B. Bulk Mail | C. Direct Mail, Office News-letters | D. News-paper | E. Allied Health Profes-sional Referral | F. Local Cable TV, Radio |
|---|---|---|---|---|---|---|
| Marketing cost | $600 | $800 | $960 | $1,008 | $750 | $2,000 |
| Number of phone inquiries | 40 | 52 | 12 | 30 | 8 | 20 |
| Number of patients realized: |  |  |  |  |  |  |
| General | 15 | 18 | 6 | 12 | 6 | 12 |
| Specialty | 5 | 12 | 4 | 8 | 2 | 3 |
| Number of products dispensed: |  |  |  |  |  |  |
| Spectacles | 10 | 14 | 4 | 9 | 6 | 10 |
| Contact lenses | 5 | 8 | 4 | 6 | 2 | 2 |
| Gross revenue: |  |  |  |  |  |  |
| Services | $1,000 | $1,500 | $500 | $1,000 | $400 | $750 |
| Products | $2,000 | $2,200 | $900 | $1,950 | $1,100 | $1,700 |
| Total | $3,000 | $3,700 | $1,400 | $2,950 | $1,500 | $2,450 |

Explanation of marketing tactics cost:

A. *Yellow Pages.* For a small display ad, the annual cost is $2,400; therefore, the quarterly cost is $600.

B. *Bulk Mail Coupon.* For example, Val-Pak, Super Coups, or Money Mailers cost about $400 per 10,000 residences per mailing. The office contract is for mailing to 20,000 residencies four times per year; therefore, the quarterly cost is $400 × 2 = $800.

C. *Direct Mail Newsletter.* The office performs quarterly bulk mailing to 2,000 computer-generated patient labels at a cost of $0.48 per address; therefore, 2,000 × $.48 = $960.

D. *Print Media.* An eighth-page display ad appears in the local weekly newspaper at a cost of $84.00 per issue × 12 weeks = $1,008 per quarter.

E. *Allied Health Care Professional Referral.* You've developed an eight-page office brochure detailing services offered and personal qualifications mailed out to all 200 dentists, physicians, osteopaths, chiropractors, and other health professionals in your area at a one-time cost of $750 for production and postage.

F. *Local Cable TV and Radio.* Usually expensive, first-time advertisers can often negotiate limited trial-period programs at reduced rates. The TV and radio companies assume all costs.

To achieve the best possible results from the use of the tracking table, it is essential that your office be as diligent as possible in obtaining the source from which the patient was referred. Staff members have at least three opportunities during the patient encounter to obtain this information. With such information, you can track the number of patients to the specific marketing option that brought them to the practice.

The first opportunity surfaces with telephone conversation when the initial appointment is made. Your receptionist can simply inquire with a casual comment, such as "By the way, how did you hear about our office?" A slightly more formal approach could be "Our office is conducting an informal in-house phone survey for the purpose of offering increased services. Could you tell us how you were referred to our facilities?" Should this first encounter prove unsuccessful, due to an oversight by your staff or the patient's inability to remember "when put on the spot," then a second opportunity to obtain the needed information can be found on the New Patient Information form completed on a patient's first visit. This can be as simple as a one-line question: "Where did you find out about our office?" A more direct approach could list all the options you are tracking. Table 6–9 illustrates this method. The advantage of listing the specific marketing options may make it easier for a patient to remember than open-ended questions. The third opportunity to identify the referral source comes during the patient's exam. You can casually ask, "By

**Table 6–9   Referral Source Questionnaire**

Please check off from the choices below how you found out about our office.

| | |
|---|---|
| Newspaper Advertisement | _____ |
| Direct Mail Coupon | _____ |
| Phone Book/Yellow Pages | _____ |
| Office Newsletter | _____ |
| Referred by Health Care Professional | _____ |
| Cable TV/Radio | _____ |
| Other | _____ |

the way, how did you hear about our office?" From the response, additional comments or discussion could arise, if desired. This is a great opportunity to find out the identity of patients referring others to your office.

There are sufficient opportunities for monitoring the source of patient referrals. This essential feedback must be collected to properly evaluate the effectiveness of all marketing tactics used. If not, then unsuccessful programs may continue and successful ones may be given only a one-time opportunity.

### Optional Tracking Method

The previous example was simplified for illustrative purposes; however, more columns can be added, depending on the number of tactics you wish to track. Other sources of patient referrals that can be monitored include former patients, nonmedical or business referrals, community civic group relations, and speaking engagements. Table 6–8 gives the gross revenue in dollars each program yields shown in the bottom row. A more precise figure can be calculated if four more rows are added on the bottom, as shown in Table 6–10: COGS (cost of goods sold), Gross profit, Marketing cost (which is the same as in Table 6–8), and Net profit. In this method, only the variable costs specifically associated with each product or service are added. We assume the fixed

**Table 6–10    Additional Cost-Profit Calculations**

|  | A. Yellow Pages | B. Bulk Mail | C. Direct Mail, Office News- letters | D. News- paper | E. Allied Health Profes- sional Referral | F. Local Cable TV, Radio |
|---|---|---|---|---|---|---|
| Total gross revenue | $3,000 | $3,700 | $1,400 | $2,950 | $1,500 | $2,450 |
| COGS | –$800 | –$1,100 | –$300 | –$700 | –$400 | $0 |
| Gross profit | $2,200 | $2,600 | $1,100 | $2,250 | $1,100 | $2,450 |
| Marketing cost (from Table 6–8) | –$600 | –$800 | –$960 | –$1,008 | –$750 | –$2,000 |
| Net profit | $1,600 | $1,800 | $240 | $1,242 | $350 | $450 |

office costs will be the same for any marketing tactic undertaken. Gross profit is the amount each program yields less the added variable costs that program produces. Net profit is determined by subtracting the marketing costs from gross profit.

A quick review of Tables 6–8 and 6–10 can be quite informative. For example, should the number of patients realized be less than 60% of the phone inquiries received, you may have a problem with your telephone reception area. The initiation of a telephone protocol to increase the percentage of new patients realized may prove beneficial. In addition, you must decide what is the minimum acceptable return on investment to continue a particular program. This will vary greatly and the opportunity cost of implementing one program must be weighed against another. Certain options may produce less dramatic but always guaranteed consistent results (which practitioners might prefer) and thus justify continuation of that marketing choice.

A survey of 421 health care providers asked what methods of marketing they most preferred.[28] Table 6–11 lists the order of preference of the various methods. Comparing the current results to the same survey taken five years earlier showed a significant increase in those providers that ask patients for referrals while Yellow Pages dipped slightly. Another marketing option on the rise, charity-related marketing, was cited in Table 1–2. A survey by Cone/Roper of 2,000 adults found that 76% had a "very or

**Table 6–11    Preferred Marketing Methods (most to least)**

1. Asking patients for referrals
2. Yellow Pages
3. Community activities
4. Ask colleagues for referrals
5. Newspaper
6. Direct mail
7. Religious-affiliated activities
8. Other print ads
9. Radio
10. Website

somewhat acceptable" opinion of this form of marketing.[29] If you decide to undergo a charity-related marketing campaign, choosing causes relevant to your practice, eyecare, or have personal meaning and local awareness is suggested. Do not abandon the marketing prematurely; be selective and diplomatic about the way you present this topic to patients, because some causes will have little appeal to certain demographic groups.[17] Table 6–12 shows an example of a monthly marketing calendar that an ECP can develop. This is one way of implementing a variety of marketing tactics each year while eliminating those that have not been successful.

**Table 6–12    Marketing Promotional Tactics Calendar**

| Month | Marketing Tactic Activity |
| --- | --- |
| January | Review telephone scripts<br>Update practice brochure<br>Mail first-quarter newsletter, promoting specialty eyewear for VDT users<br>Plan Valentine's Day promotion<br>Send letter to local pediatricians and PCPs |
| February | Send Save Your Vision Week (SYVW) materials and news release to local schools<br>Send Valentine's Day cards statement stuffer: "Is your loved one overdue for an eye exam?"<br>Show "A Journey Through Your Eyes" video at local elementary schools<br>Offer to host tours of office for class field trip<br>Have frame reps do in-office presentations for staff |
| March | Speak to local PTAs on "Vision and Learning"<br>Include SYVW reminder in monthly billings<br>Have office special on colored or special contact lenses<br>Review pretesting scripts with technicians<br>Mail out annual patient satisfaction survey |
| April | Speak to local civic groups on "Allergies and Your Eyes"<br>Send out direct mailing to companies with VDT workers<br>Mail second-quarter newsletter. Possible topics: Don't forget spare CLs for vacation, summer eye safety (fireworks, summer sports, UV protection), children's annual eye exams. |

*(continues)*

**Table 6–12  (Continued)**

| *Month* | *Marketing Tactic Activity* |
|---|---|
| May | Free blood pressure screenings for all patients<br>Special on summer eyewear and accessories<br>Prepare Mother's Day cards for mailing<br>Press release on UV dangers sent to local papers<br>Participate in AARP's 55 Alive driving clinic<br>New presbyopic options brochure sent to patients age 40–60 |
| June | Special on progressive lenses<br>Father's Day special<br>Press release on dangers of fireworks sent to local papers<br>Contact local library to supply displays for summer reading program |
| July | Review lens option demonstration scripts<br>Workshop for coaches on "Sports Vision Training"<br>Mail third-quarter newsletter. Topics: Back-to-school exams for students, prescription drugs and vision, Medicare Q&A |
| August | Have an open house on one Saturday<br>Send "ABC's of Eyecare Vision Guides for Teachers" to local schools<br>Vision care mailing to school nurses<br>Sports vision screening for local school athletic teams |
| September | Occupational vision and safety screening for factory workers<br>Offer public relations workshop at community college or civic group |
| October | Develop marketing plan calendar for next year<br>Speak to local civic groups on "Warning Signs of Vision Problems"<br>Send press release to local newspaper on "Hazards of Limited Vision in Halloween Costumes"<br>Mail fourth-quarter newsletter. Topics: Eyecare for diabetics, eyewear and accessories for Christmas, dangers of eye injury from children's toys, protective eyewear for winter sports |
| November | Glaucoma, cataract, and diabetic retinopathy screenings at nursing homes<br>Mailing to patients known to be diabetic<br>Special offer to veterans<br>Special on 100% UV-protective sports eyewear<br>Send press release on dangerous toys to local newspapers |
| December | Newsletter and newspaper article on suggested toys for different age groups and toys dangerous to children's vision<br>Promote vision safety with PTA's, Lion's Clubs, churches<br>Finalize next year's marketing plan calendar |

## Strategies for Increasing the Number of Referrals from PCPs

Many ECPs have been successful in receiving referrals from primary care physicians (PCP) while others are less successful. Appendix 6–3 lists strategies to increase the number of referrals from this potentially lucrative source. ECPs are in an ideal position to refer patients to general physicians. General physicians typically will not refer patients to other general physicians that are competitors. Specialists do not refer patients because the patient already has a PCP to get to the specialist. Many eyecare patients, however, do not seek routine medical care. Some physicians say ECPs refer more patients to them than anyone else. These physicians like working with ECPs. The following is a list of suggestions for an ECP to implement when starting a PCP referral program.

1. Use questions in your history form that may lead to a referral: Who is your general physician? When was the last time you had a physical? Do you have any of the following symptoms?

2. When reviewing the history with the patients, ask if they are happy with their general physician. If not, offer to introduce them to one you work with. One ECP will walk the patient across the hall to a physician and introduce the patient as a friend. "Hello, Bill. This is my friend, Ms. Gaines. She is looking for a new physician. I told her you are the best. Please take good care of her." Other ECPs will pick up the telephone and call: "Bill, I've got a patient here who I think you will enjoy. I'm sending Ms. Gaines over to meet you. I know you will take good care of her." By asking patients if they are happy with their PCPs, you learn which ones are best to be associated with.

3. Following your examination, you may wish to encourage your patient to seek a general physical examination. "Ms. Gaines, I can take good care of your eyes, and you seem to be healthy physically. However, you have not had a physical in 3 years. I'd like to make an appointment for you with Dr.

Stoner. He is an excellent doctor. It is a good idea for a physician to get to know you before you have a problem."

4. Include procedures in your examination that may lead to referrals. Take blood pressure, look for signs of elevated cholesterol, diabetes, discuss feelings of general fatigue, and signs of depression. "Ms. Gaines, your blood pressure is a little high today. I do not see any signs of problems in your eyes related to the high blood pressure, but I'd like a physical examination to ensure you take steps to keep it under control. Dr. Stoner is an internist who specializes in high blood pressure. Here is a biographical sketch about him. I'd like to have Mary make an appointment for you now. If he has any questions, have him give me a call."

5. Ask the PCPs you are targeting to send patient education materials to assist in making referrals. This can include business cards, biographical sketches, brochures, pamphlets about medical conditions, and videotapes about medical conditions. By developing a referral line to the PCP you are setting the stage for receiving referrals.

**Marketing Directed at Your Personal PCP**

A good physician to begin with is your own family physician. If you receive no referrals from him or her, it may be best to change physicians. Thank your physician for his or her help and offer a free eye examination and spectacles at cost. Call and make the appointment then or at the end of that day. Tell the doctor you will forward information of interest on physical conditions and medications that may result in vision problems. According to Robert Crawford, O.D., of Brockton, Massachusetts, "once you show the MDs what you can do, the referrals will be never-ending. There are tremendous opportunities in this area. O.D.s just need to get out, 'pound the pavement' a little, connect with medical groups, and be aggressive; they will like what we can do."[30]

**Market to the Patient's PCP**

6. Send an examination summary to the PCP after every eye examination.

7. Tell the PCP when you wish to examine his or her patient again.
8. Include a peel-off sticker to be placed in the patient's file with the next scheduled appointment.

## Educate PCPs on What ECPs Do

9. Write letters highlighting diagnosis and treatment.
10. Invite PCP for tour of the office.
11. Give free examinations, offer courtesy to family members.
12. Copy articles on systemic conditions and their effects on vision.
13. Visit PCPs' offices and invite them to join your referral network; ask for cards, brochures, biographical sketches.
14. Provide the PCP with business cards, brochures, and biographical sketches.
15. Call the PCP for referral to retinal specialist. Develop a script that impresses the PCP on your knowledge.

## Develop Personal Relationships with PCPs

Stop and think for a moment. To whom are you apt to refer someone who requires assistance outside the health care field? Perhaps you know someone who requires an insurance agent or a golf professional. To whom would you refer them? Most of us give referrals to friends in the business.

16. By becoming a "friend" with physicians, marketing, educating, and enhancing referrals become easier. Develop a personal relationship with physicians. Play golf, tennis, participate in church activities, create friendships between wives and children. Lunch together, vacation together. People refer to friends. Find common interests and build on them.
17. If for some reason you cannot, then perhaps your spouse or a staff member will be able to build a relationship.

## Market to the PCP's Staff

Many ECPs find it much easier to build referral relationships with a physician's staff member. Staff members often write most of the referrals from managed care plans. The nurse, receptionist, or office manager may respond to friendly interaction, whereas the physician is too busy. How often do you suppose overworked staff members are treated to free meals and entertainment? Is it common for staff members to complain of lack of recognition? As ECPs, we can give them recognition, either alone or with our staffs.

18. By having a regular lunch or giving a free eye exam, you can learn about how the managed care referrals work within the PCP's office. Work with the office staff to make referrals easier for them. A typical problem with so many managed care plans is that the PCP staff members do not know to whom to send their patients. One ECP says, "Send all your managed care patients to us. We will then assist them in finding the ECP who can examine them under their plan." This action assists the PCP staff with a problem and puts you in control of who the patient sees.

### Thank PCP Offices for Referrals

19. Send a thank you note or express your appreciation in a manner that the referring PCP and staff would find appropriate. People like to be thanked. This will encourage more referrals. Staff members, in particular, like to feel appreciated.

### Consider Hospital Privileges

20. Gaining hospital privileges will provide you with more opportunities to interact with physicians and allow you to educate them. Sometimes, Independent Provider Associations are unable to refer patients to you unless you are on the hospital-based IPA. This often requires you to have hospital privileges. Hospitals may have telephone referral services. You may not be included on the referral list unless you have hospital privileges. Gaining hospital privileges may require a great deal of personal networking and lobbying. Hospitals often require donations of time and money from their staff providers, which must be factored into the appeal of being on staff.

Primary care physicians are similar to ECPs in many ways. They are overworked, confused with managed care, and often have little time to deal with issues outside their immediate needs. There is very little reason for PCPs to be motivated about learning what ECPs can do for them. Therefore, you must take the initiative and develop plans to encourage referrals from PCP offices. Target a physician, look over the preceding strategies used by ECPs, develop a plan, and be consistent. Put yourself in the PCP's position. What would encourage you, as a ECP, to refer to the optometrist in town? Relate this answer to a specific PCP's attitude and personality, and you are on your way to building referrals.

## Patient Expectations

When developing your four *P*'s marketing mix, take into account the patient's point of view and consider the four Cs.[31] As the seller you are going to *promote* your *products* (and services) using predetermined *prices* at a specific *place* (your office). Your patients, however, expect to receive *customer value* at an acceptable *cost* and *convenient* location that they will find out about through your various marketing *communications*.

Two components of the marketing mix have a tremendous influence on the image you present to your patients: the communication methods you use in your promotions and the pricing strategy you choose for your products and services. The way you communicate with your patients falls into two categories: those over which you have little or no control (word of mouth and patient needs) and those you can influence (advertising, point-of-purchase materials, personal selling, and those aspects of the patient visit pertaining to the appearance of the office and staff). Price also influences patient expectations. Patients who lack information about the quality of a service you offer often substitute price as a replacement for quality.[32] Prices set too low may send signals that the services you offer are of little value or low quality, while prices set too high may be difficult to justify or cause patients to develop expectations that are difficult for the practice to meet.

Expectations are the baseline against which patients evaluate performance. **You can influence patient expectations through patient perceptions by altering the marketing mix through com-**

munication programs, pricing strategy, and continually monitoring the quality of your products and services to establish the highest possible standards of performance. This knowledge is critical to determining and understanding patient satisfaction.

## Action Plan for ECPs

1. Identify your core competencies.
2. Determine what specific parts of your practice systems and operations contribute to the value your patients desire.
3. Where can you enhance the value chain to offer your patients increased benefits?
4. Recognize how you presently use each of the four *P*s to market your practice and how you could alter what you are doing to improve your results. Complete the Fee Strategy Checklist (Appendix 6–1).
5. Complete the Additional Marketing Tactics checklist (Appendix 6–2) and combine the results with Marketing During the Patient Visit (Appendix 5–3) to determine the optimal marketing mix for your present situation.
6. Complete the Generating Referrals from Primary Care Physicians questionnaire (Appendix 6–3) and add the results to your marketing mix.
7. Develop a draft Marketing Promotional Tactics Calendar similar to that in Table 6–12.
8. Initiate a short-term tracking system using three or four different promotional techniques using Tables 6–8 and 6–10.
9. Apply the marketing Dos and Don'ts shown in Table 6–13 to your particular situation.

**Table 6–13   Marketing Dos and Don'ts**

1. Do anticipate the response requirements and patient retention needs.
2. Do track results to determine the most cost-effective methods of marketing.
3. Do analyze the consequences of leaving plans to potential present and future patient loss.
4. Don't copycat your competitor's marketing; this decreases your ability to differentiate your practice.
5. Don't retrench immediately if results are taking longer than projected.

# Fee Strategy Checklist

Here is a checklist of fee strategies. Check those strategies you're using now. Next, put a check in the second column for three pricing changes that you would like to try.

| Strategy | Do Now | Want to Try |
|---|---|---|
| 1. Give a courtesy discount when a family schedules two or more eye exams within a month. | | |
| 2. Give a courtesy discount when an individual or family orders two or more pairs of glasses or contacts at one time. | | |
| 3. Accept major credit cards. | | |
| 4. Accept insurance assignment. | | |
| 5. Develop employee plans with major employers in your area. | | |
| 6. Offer payment plans with no interest. | | |
| 7. Require deposits or payment in full on frames, lenses, or contacts. | | |
| 8. Offer preseason prices, such as discounts on sunglasses or ski goggles, at the appropriate times of the year. | | |
| 9. Find out which employers cover vision care services. | | |
| 10. Offer repairs or adjustments with no additional cost | | |
| On all eyewear. | | |
| Only on eyewear obtained through your dispensary. | | |
| 11. Offer financing at a fixed-percent interest. | | |
| 12. Arrange outside financing. | | |

| Strategy | Do Now | Want to Try |
|---|---|---|
| 13. Offer a courtesy discount | | |
| to other health care providers. | | |
| to their friends or staff. | | |
| to their family. | | |
| 16. Other (specify) | | |

# Additional Marketing Tactics to Use in Your Office

Review the following list of tactics and decide which you believe would be the most effective as part of your marketing mix.

| Marketing Technique | Using Success- fully | Using but Needs Im- provement | Not Using but Want To | Not Appro- priate |
|---|---|---|---|---|
| Marketing prior to starting the business | | | | |
| Marketing plan | | | | |
| Survey | | | | |
| Identity or image | | | | |
| Name | | | | |
| Theme | | | | |
| Niche | | | | |
| Logo | | | | |
| Quality | | | | |
| Pricing | | | | |
| Selection | | | | |
| Marketing to bring in new patients | | | | |
| Direct mail | | | | |
| Demographics research | | | | |
| Newspaper inserts | | | | |
| Refrigerator magnets | | | | |
| Newspaper ads | | | | |
| Courses and lectures | | | | |

| Marketing Technique | Using Success-fully | Using but Needs Im-provement | Not Using but Want To | Not Appro-priate |
|---|---|---|---|---|
| School in-service | | | | |
| Seminars | | | | |
| Trunk shows | | | | |
| Medical practitioner referrals | | | | |
| Contests | | | | |
| Scholarships and awards | | | | |
| Community activities | | | | |
| Public relations | | | | |
| Club and associations | | | | |
| Outside signs | | | | |
| Reputation | | | | |
| Word of mouth | | | | |
| Tie-in with other professionals | | | | |
| Co-op funding | | | | |
| Radio ads and shows | | | | |
| Television ads and shows | | | | |
| Magazine ads and articles | | | | |
| Billboards | | | | |
| *Marketing convenience as a benefit to the patient* | | | | |
| Availability of financing | | | | |
| Credit cards accepted | | | | |
| ATM payment | | | | |
| Courtesy billing | | | | |
| Courtesy discounts | | | | |
| Hours of operation | | | | |
| Days of operation | | | | |
| Free consultations | | | | |
| Speed | | | | |
| Schedule over the Internet | | | | |

| Marketing Technique | Using Successfully | Using but Needs Improvement | Not Using but Want To | Not Appropriate |
|---|---|---|---|---|
| Order over the Internet | | | | |
| Patient pickup and return | | | | |
| Home delivery of products | | | | |
| Website information | | | | |

# Generating Referrals from Primary Care Physicians

The expansion of the scope of eyecare practice combined with managed care has enhanced the need for working together with primary care physicians. The questions here cover 20 ways ECPs can use to develop relationships with primary care physicians that will result in referrals.

1. Do you refer patients to the primary care physicians?
   a. What patient history questions do you ask that generate referrals to a PCP?
   b. Do you review the PCP's history with the patient?
   c. What test procedures lead to referrals?
   d. During your case summary, how do you present your exam results and make recommendations?
   e. Do you use patient education materials educating the patient about the physician and their medical condition?
2. Do you market your practice to your personal or family MD?
3. When you market to the patient's PCP do you supply examination summaries and ask for summary results of their exam?
4. How do you educate PCPs on what you do?
   a. Letters?
   b. Tour of the office?
   c. Free examinations, courtesy to family members?
   d. Articles on systemic conditions that affect vision?
   e. Visit their offices?
   f. Invite them to join your referral network?
   g. Provide the PCP materials that tell about you?
   h. Call the PCP for referral to retinal specialists?

5. How do you develop relationships with physicians with whom you have common interests?
   a. Personally?
   b. Through your spouse?
   c. Through a staff member?
6. Do you market to PCP's staff members by inviting them to
   a. Lunch?
   b. Free eye exams?
7. Do you thank the PCP and the office staff for the referral with both a phone call and a follow-up letter?
8. Have you attempted or succeeded in obtaining hospital privileges?
9. When was the last time you referred a friend to a specific PCP? Why did you choose that person?
10. Why should a PCP refer patients to you instead of another eyecare practitioner?
11. How much does it cost to give a free eye exam if you have an appointment slot open?
12. What can you do for the staff in a PCP's office to encourage referrals?

# Notes

1. Porter M. *Competitive Advantage: Creating and Sustaining Superior Performance.* New York: Free Press; 1985.
2. Borden N. Concept of the marketing mix. Harvard Business School case no. 9-502-004, 1962.
3. Borden N. The concept of the marketing mix. In: Schwartz G, ed. *Science in Marketing.* New York: John Wiley; 1965:386–397.
4. Maves G. "Better measures for direct marketing. *Marketing.* October 3, 1991:32.
5. Perrault W, McCarthy E. *Basic Marketing,* 13th ed. Boston: Irwin McGraw-Hill; 1999:47.
6. Kent R. Faith in the four Ps: An alternative. *Journal of Marketing Management.* 1986;2(2):145–154.
7. Booms B, Bitner M. Marketing strategies and organization structure for service firms. In: Donnelly J, George W, eds. *Marketing of Services.* Chicago: American Marketing Association; 1981:47–51.
8. Brookes R. *The New Marketing.* Aldershot, England: Gower Press; 1988.
9. Bennett P. *Dictionary of Marketing Terms.* Chicago: American Marketing Association; 1988:21.
10. Shostack GL, Kingman-Brundage J. Service design and development. In: Congram C, Friedman M, *Handbook of Services Marketing.* New York: American Management Association, 1990.
11. Graham J. How much should a company spend on marketing? *American Salesman.* June 1995;40(6):13–15.
12. Massnick F. Customer service can kill you. *Management Review.* March 1997;86(3):33–35.
13. Sturm A. *The New Rules of Healthcare Marketing.* Chicago: Health Administration Press; 1998:50.
14. Winston G. "How to get the most bang for your marketing bucks. *American Banker.* June 16, 1994;159(115):27.
15. Study reveals crucial sales tips. *Genesis Training Solutions.* [Genesis, 23 Skyland Pl., The Woodlands, TX 77381].
16. D. Howard. Survey of successful marketing tactics, July 25, 2000.

17. Horrocks W, Pinton W. *Unlimited New Patients.* Washington, DC: New Patients, Inc.; 1994.
18. Medical Group Management. Proven methods for cross-selling services. *Marketer's Guidepost.* November–December 1996;7(6):1.
19. S. Sokol. Internet survey ascertaining factors of success. July 27, 2000.
20. Miscall R. Pick a card. *Denver Business Journal.* October 23 1998;50(8):17–18.
21. Lohse G. Consumer eye movement patterns on yellow pages. *Journal of Advertising.* Spring 1997;26(1):61–73.
22. Chesanow N. How one group builds market leadership. *Medical Economics.* February 23, 1998;75(4):92.
23. Solomon R. *The Physician Manager's Handbook.* Gaithersburg, MD: Aspen Publishers; 1997:256.
24. Reading N. Setting practice fees. *Medical Practice Management.* January–February 2000;15(4):200-202.
25. Berry L, Parasuraman A. *Marketing Services.* New York: Free Press; 1991:101–102.
26. Corey R. Marketing strategy—An overview. Harvard Business School case no. 9-579-054, 1992.
27. Moss G. Monitored marketing. *Optometric Economics.* July 1994;4(7):26–28.
28. Patient referrals rank as doctors' #1 marketing option. *Dental Practice and Finance.* September–October 1999:6.
29. Barner C. Giving back. *Dental Practice and Finance.* July–August 1999:48–52.
30. R. Crawford, e-mail, Survey of successful marketing tactics, July 25, 2000.
31. Lautenborn R. New marketing litany: 4P's passé; c-words takeover. *Advertising Age.* October 1, 1990:26.
32. Clarke B, Sucher T. Benchmarking for the competitive marketplace. *Journal of Ambulatory Care Management.* July 1999; 22(3):72–78.

## CHAPTER 7

# Understanding Patient Satisfaction

> The only real way to distinguish yourself from the competition is through service.
>
> —*John Tisch*[1]

A survey reported in the *Harvard Business Review* showed that American business leaders rank customer satisfaction and product quality as the two highest priorities ultimately influencing the success of their organizations.[2] A complementary study performed by the market research firm Michaelson & Associates reported that poor service and product dissatisfaction were the two primary reasons why customers would not return to a retail operation.[3] The ECP with a goal of delivering the highest possible level of patient satisfaction always faces two challenges: first, patients' uncertainty about how genuine they perceive your concern; second, despite superior quality, patient dissatisfaction due to personality conflicts or staff unfriendliness.

One survey of service quality showed that 40% of consumers change to the competition because of poor *perceived* service, while only 8% change because of price.[4] This survey reported it was five times less expensive and easier to keep an existing client than recruit a new one. Another study suggests that it costs 10 times more to convince a dissatisfied customer to return.[5] The U.S. Office of Consumer Affairs reports that a dissatisfied customer will tell at least nine additional people about his or her dissatisfaction, which makes sacrificing a good reputation much faster than gaining a favorable one.[6] All these observations are affected by the daily business decisions ECPs make. The evidence supports directing marketing efforts toward current patients and making sure patients do not leave your office dissatisfied.

Studies show high-quality service is more effective at increasing both volume of business and levels of profitability in certain business settings than advertising and promotions.[7] There are many ways to enhance the marketing capabilities of any business. Here are seven recommendations to serve as a guide when developing a marketing program directly related to producing patient satisfaction:[8]

1. Patients do not buy your services, they buy *solutions* to their problems.
2. High-quality service delivery means never saying "that's not my responsibility."
3. How you and your staff feel eventually is how your patient will feel.
4. Patients should never have to complain more than once before the problem is resolved.
5. If you establish negative expectations for your patients, you always will meet them.
6. The delivery of high-quality service is never the patient's job.
7. If you are the underdog, avoid head-to-head competition, target segments where you can offer specialized services that allow you to emphasize your strengths.

## Service Quality

The distinction in levels of quality of business performance were first made apparent by Dr. Walter Shewhart, working for Bell Laboratories in the 1920s. He applied statistical charting to determine differences between "controlled" and "uncontrolled" variations in the work process.[9] This concept was taken further by one of Shewhart's students, W. E. Deming, who worked with him prior to World War II. Deming along with J. M. Duran developed what was to become known as *total quality management.*

Many researchers have attempted to define the parameters of high-quality service businesses provide to patrons, but in essence, "service quality is the foundation for services marketing because the core product being marketed is performance. The performance is the product; the performance is what customers buy."[10] The perception developed by patients always poses a potential risk, and "customer's perception of risk tends to be high for services because services cannot be touched, smelled, tasted or tried on before purchase."[11]

The ability to differentiate one practice from another is a marketing advantage the ECP gains as an added benefit by delivering consistently reliable service. **This results in higher patient retention, decreased spending on new patient recruitment, increased word-of-mouth advertising, and greater opportunity to charge higher fees.** When it comes to high-quality care, patients want what they expect, and if delivered, they will be satisfied, a key component of patient loyalty and retention. From the standpoint of employee morale, a high-quality experience for patients results in higher levels of motivation, morale, job satisfaction, and commitment—all found to be inversely related to their daily experiences with patient frustration levels.[8]

## Measuring Quality

"Credentialling" and "report carding" are relatively new topics in the ophthalmic profession. However, increasingly, both ECPs and third-party payers are concerned about "economic credentialling and the impact that the focus on money will have on the quality of health care."[3] Neither Health Care Finance Administration (HCFA) nor the U.S. government has yet to identify a specific system to use for either report cards or ratings, but methods have appeared on the Internet, such as www.Healthcarereportcards.com.[3] In addition, the National Committee for Quality Assurance created the "Quality Compass," a database of quality indicators. Finally, the latest version of the Health Plan Employer Data Information Set (HEDIS) 3.4 includes clinical as well as member satisfaction data.

How do you reach the goal of offering the highest possible service quality? One way is to instill, as part of your practice culture, a zero-defect service delivery mindset. This requires your office performance to be error free during the initial patient visit. Next, you must understand the patient's expectations and requirements, because these establish the critical standards against which your performance is evaluated. Finally, recognize that, even when you deliver "perfectly accurate" service or products, patients may perceive it as flawed if they become confused or frustrated. How many times have you had a patient receive a first pair of progressive-add lenses just to return them in two to three days telling you the new glasses are "wrong"? Your investigation of the patient's complaint reveals that the problem is not in the fabrication but rather in the improper way the patient has been adapting to and using the glasses. In this case, inadequate information was given to the patient. Satisfaction with the information given has been proposed as a necessary component of overall customer satisfaction.[12]

A direct advantage of providing superior service is added revenue, a claim supported by a Wall Street Journal/NBC News survey, confirming that consumers are willing to pay higher prices for superior service.[13] The survey revealed that 35% of the respondents stated they would purchase more expensive services as long as they believed the business provides better service. An additional 40% said that, at least part of the time, they would purchase higher-priced but better services. This is the belief of Ron Seger, O.D., of Mountain View, CA, who states, "We always make a point of advising each patient that they are a candidate for contact lenses. . . . Most patients with 0.75 cylinder or more will chose to be fitted with soft toric contact lenses. . . . This is the ultimate win-win situation. The patient sees better, because you have provided a higher level of service and took the time to communicate an option that was potentially better for their eyes. . . . The doctor is able to charge more. . . . Satisfied patients will tell their friends about what a great job you did for them."[14]

## RATER

The following five main characteristics of service delivery that contribute to patients' overall perceptions about quality are referred to as RATER:[15]

1. *Reliability.* The ability to perform the promised service dependably and accurately.
2. *Assurance.* The staff's knowledge, courtesy, and ability to convey credibility, trustworthiness, and competence.
3. *Tangibles.* The physical appearance of facility, equipment, staff, and communication materials.
4. *Empathy.* Caring, individualized attention; understanding patient's concerns, situation, and communication.
5. *Responsiveness.* Willingness to assist patients and provide prompt service without patient experiencing obstacles or an inability to gain access to your services.

Of the five stated components of service quality, reliability is an outcome, while the other four are part of the service delivery process; the last three often are a direct result of employee performance.[16] Studies performed over the past 15 years in a variety of settings confirm that "evidence from our research consistently shows that reliability is the foremost criterion customers consider in evaluating a company's quality of service."[15]

How do you utilize the characteristics of RATER to achieve higher levels of patient satisfaction, leading to patient loyalty and retention? An extensive study, in 1997, the Service Oriented Accredited Research, identified areas of existing differences between the beliefs of providers and patients.[17] Of the five components of RATER, tangibles, empathy, and assurance were perceived to be the same by both provider and patient. Tangibles are concerned with the cleanliness of the office and staff personnel. Empathy considers the amount of individual attention each patient is given. Assurance is achieved by the provider and staff displaying a warm, friendly, open demeanor toward patient. The fourth attribute of RATER, responsiveness, was believed by providers to be achieved by listening to and answering patient's questions, while patients felt it was better displayed by the staff's and provider's willingness to accommodate and respond to the patient's particular needs. The fifth and most important component of achieving patient satisfaction, reliability, had the greatest variety of attributes. A myriad of factors, including no mistakes, repeatability, efficiency, and timeliness, are components of both the patient's and provider's concepts of reliability. Providers believed promptness and adhering to scheduled appointments led to satisfaction, while patients felt that error-free records, clinical and financial, were predominant factors in achieving reliable service and patient satisfaction. Even the federal government is sensitive to this issue, as is evident by the U.S. Senate's introduction, in April 2000, of the Stop All Frequent Errors in Medicare and Medicaid Act.[18]

One conclusion drawn from these similarities and differences in the qualities of RATER is that providers should concentrate on demonstrating what patients perceive most easily, not always what the provider believes patients want or need. Another important finding supported by research is that, of patients who rate their provider as "excellent," 85% recommend that provider to other people, but only 50% of patients claiming to have received "very good care" refer their provider to someone else. Only 10% of patients who believed they received "good care" recommend their provider.[19] **Therefore, it is not enough to simply do a good job if you want patients to be advocates of your practice. To produce enthusiastic patients who readily recommend your office requires you deliver consistently excellent service in the opinion of your patients.** If you want patients to promote your practice, you could infer that, in the health care industry, "good is not good enough" and only "delighted" patients exhibit the necessary enthusiasm to produce a successful word-of-mouth campaign.[20]

Consider the following application of RATER in the eyecare setting:[21]

- If you fulfill a patient's order on time, you are showing that your services are reliable.
- If your staff smiles and tells patients that they would like to help them, your practice is building assurance.
- If you take time to make yourself and your office presentable, you are showing concern for the tangible.
- If you display sensitivity when resolving patient problems, you are demonstrating empathy.
- When you offer advice to a patient that seems distressed, you are showing responsiveness.

## Patient Satisfaction

Intuitively, it is reasonable to expect that a satisfied customer, in most instances, will spend more than a dissatisfied customer. In fact, this has been substantiated by a Technical Assistance Research Project study in Washington, D.C., which showed the accounts of customers reporting service satisfaction were three times more profitable than those unsatisfied.[22] As one extensive study reported, depending on the industry, a reduction of just 5% in customer attrition can result in profit increases of 25–85%.[23] Another authority claims that increasing patient retention by 2% can decrease practice costs by up to 10%.[24] However, it is not simply gaining added revenue where patient satisfaction becomes an important issue. Another compelling reason to strive for patient satisfaction is found in the area of risk management. Extensive research has found that three quarters of all health care-related lawsuits arise from patients feeling they were mistreated.[25]

Always take into account the patients' wants, needs, and their criteria to produce patient satisfaction. Another view of patient satisfaction with health care providers is expressed through an understanding of consumerism. Regina Herzlinger, professor of health care economics at Harvard Business School, proposes that the patient, as consumer, has three requirements that must be met in order to be satisfied:[26] convenience, control, and ability to freely choose whom to see, accompanied by the information necessary to make an informed choice concerning the three criteria. A different source suggests that the perception of quality patients develop may be influenced by the level of caring, professionalism, and competence they receive from your staff.[27] **To date, no single theory encompasses all the requirements to produce patient satisfaction a majority of the time; therefore, you can benefit from an understanding of several theories on satisfaction.**

### Patient Satisfaction versus Perceived Service Quality

Presently there are two theories that dominate the discussions relevant to customer satisfaction. The first is the comparison-level theory, which states that the basis for the decision a customer makes to remain loyal is the "lowest level of outcomes a person will accept in light of available alternative opportunities."[28] This is based on the patient's perception of what the competition offers. The second theory is known as the disconfirmation of expectancy paradigm.[29] Simply put, **satisfaction is the difference between the patient's previsit expectations in relation to the cost they incur and the performance level or value he or she actually receives.** How can you favorably influence patient expectations? Educate patients by providing accurate information prior to the visit through direct mail communication or referral to the practice website. Realistic, achievable outcomes produce satisfied patients, while unrealistic, unmet outcomes result in dissatisfied patients. Professional service quality is influenced by a technical component (what the patient receives) and functional component (how it is received).[31] The technical portion is "defined primarily on the technical accuracy of the diagnosis and procedures," while the functional portion "refers to the manner in which health service is delivered to the patient."[31] Research suggests that patients are influenced more by the interpersonal, functional component of service rather than the technical components of the exam.[32]

Recent studies indicate that satisfaction with the information patients receive about a product or service they are choosing influences their level of satisfaction.[12] The quality of information given to patients becomes significant, especially if patients feel they have been misled or a product does not perform as promised, even through no fault of the ECP. This inadequate understanding of what to expect sometimes is seen with a first-time progressive addition spectacle lens patient who did not adapt well or with a first-time toric fitting, resulting in poor visual acuity due to residual astigmatism. A potential patient came into an upscale, suburban East Coast eyecare office inquiring about a specific type of specialty spectacle lens. The customer was told a price and the ophthalmic technician admitted that the lens was available for less money down the street. The customer acknowledged the technician's honesty, adding that he had just come from the other office prior to visiting this office. The patient left without making a purchase. However, the patient very likely could have been converted into a buyer by simply being given the necessary information. Educating the customer that there are different brands and levels of quality of the specialty lens desired and that this office knowingly uses a superior quality to that of the competitor would justify the higher fee. Adding the support of a longer warrantee and money-back guarantee would eliminate any doubts the customer might have about the superiority of the product to that of the competitor. Informing the patient why your product is superior, in most instances, will justify higher fees.

A survey, conducted by the Bayer Institute for Health Care Communication, revealed nearly half of patients responding believed that providers did not adequately explain what they were thinking or doing.[33] However, plans and providers typically emphasize the technical aspect of high-quality service delivery, which includes competence, processes, outcomes, and collaboration. Referring to the components of RATER discussed earlier, several recent patient focus group surveys highlight significant differences among patient, provider, and health care administrator views of delivering quality.[31] Patients did not consider clinical outcomes part of satisfaction, providers did not include courtesy, while plan administrators excluded caring. If we assume that high quality leads to satisfaction, this survey conveys what sometimes is obvious in ECP offices: **Disagreement still exists among the active participants as to how to achieve satisfaction. The only certain conclusion that can be drawn from any discussion on service quality is that "consumer preferences should be treated as absolute performance standards."[34]**

Patient satisfaction should be considered a "transitory short-term service encounter-specific perception," while the delivery of service quality is a "long-term attitude that can be operationalized by measures of service-firm performance."[35] A primary goal of achieving patient satisfaction is to positively influence a patient's purchasing intention. The sequence of events leading to this ability is shown in Figure 7–1. This diagram points out that both service quality and patient satisfaction are central components that contribute to the ECP's ability to favorably influence patient purchasing decisions.

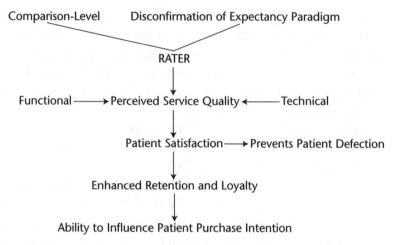

**Figure 7–1** **How service quality leads to patient satisfaction, which creates an obstacle to patient defection. The ultimate result is to enhance your ability to positively influence the patient's purchasing decision.**

## Factors That Influence the Doctor-Patient Relationship

The doctor-patient relationship is influenced by the rapport (interpersonal bond) established, the ability of the provider to allow the patient to participate in his or her own care (inclusionary bond), and the costs (monetary bond) the patient incurs.[20] A recent trend reported in a study by the Center for Studying Health System Change found that 58% of patients would be willing to accept restrictions on choice of provider in exchange for out-of-pocket savings.[36] This could give added leverage to third parties negotiating with ECPs in the future and certainly disrupt the doctor-patient relationship.

A Harris Poll survey found that the number one complaint by patients with their health care provider was the lack of timely and adequate communication from providers.[37] Another recently reported study found that **most doctors surveyed explained the nature of problems to patients, but only 9% of doctors were likely to assess the level of the patient's understanding of his or her condition.**[38] Problems also arise because patients, plans, and providers seem to have different priorities as to what should be the primary factors to emphasize when describing quality. Pa-

tients want functional quality, judging their perception of services based on courtesy, communication, understanding, responsiveness, caring, and accessibility.[20]
Four factors affect the doctor-patient relationship:[31]

1. Socioemotional elements include the perception of the provider's communication and interpersonal skills, which are functional qualities such as caring, courtesy, and empathy.
2. System-related factors include technical aspects, such as wait time, accessibility, convenience, and time spent with patient.
3. Moderating elements influence the patient's health status and needs.
4. External influencing elements include a patient's family and friends.

You should recognize the factors that affect your relationship with patients, exploiting those that strengthen the bond and compensating for those that weaken the bond.

You can apply several practical tactics to provide the highest possible service quality and strengthen the doctor-patient bond:

1. Perform in-office patient surveys and focus groups.
2. Provide customer service training to members of the staff.
3. Anticipate patient expectations, then surpass them.
4. Review and change any office systems that inconvenience patients.
5. Offer staff incentives to enhance service.
6. Focus on the functional quality of service that patients readily understand.

Evidence from researchers at the Wharton School of Business working with data from the American Customer Satisfaction Index showed that "customer loyalty is a much greater driver of profitability than even market share."[39] Studies reported in the *International Journal of Research in Marketing* showed that, even during retail sales encounters that prove to be nonproductive, perceived warmth from staff members is an indicator of perceived service quality and loyalty.[40] The implication is that, even if the patient does not make a purchase on any given occasion, the staff should not become frustrated but continue to offer a warm, likable demeanor, which in the long run will result in higher levels of patient retention. Retaining patient business in the face of increased competitive pressure requires an enterprising, adaptive provider who recognizes the benefits the practice gains through long-term patient relationships and a strong doctor-patient bond. **One guaranteed method of retaining patient loyalty is to involve the patient in "an interactive, collaborative learning relationship" that requires the patient to teach the ECP how to provide for his or her individual needs.[41] Once ECPs incorporate what the patient has taught them into their service delivery process, it becomes much more difficult for that patient to abandon that specifically unique quality of care.**

Other useful communication devices that build on the doctor-patient bond are newsletters mailed directly to patients or available while waiting in the patient lounge and postexam summary findings mailed to patients.[42] According to Donald H. Lakin, O.D., practitioner and former practice management instructor at Michigan College of Optometry

> too many health care providers believe they are "successful" when their patients have to wait three to six weeks for appointments. Although loyal patients may accept this for routine care, there is a reluctance or an indifference on their part to refer friends or other family members. New people seeking services are totally turned off and will seek services elsewhere. This type of practice will quickly lose its growth potential and will age with the practitioner. The addition of an associate doctor before the practice reaches this impacted state is critical. Availability of services on an ongoing basis is a strategy that is necessary if the practice market is going to grow. Most successful multipractitioner practices have and are using this strategy.[43]

In addition, anytime you or your staff can offer patients special, enhanced, or extraordinary services, either through added benefits or lower cost, capitalize on the opportunity to highlight what the patient has gained, because this is another way to differentiate your office from the competition. The following list offers a few opportunities of which you could take advantage:

1. *Physical setting.*[44] Make certain the surroundings are pleasant by enhancing the sights, sounds, and odors the patient experiences in your office.
2. *Interpersonal actions.* How willing are your employees to accommodate patients?
3. *Speed of service.* Don't make patients wait longer than they are willing.
4. *Cost of service.* If patients can comparison shop make sure you can justify your price.
5. *Unanticipated embellishments.* For example, coffee and *CNN Headline News* in the patient lounge.

**The standard of performance for the eyecare provider should be to fully explain, share control, seek feedback, and display concern to strengthen the doctor-patient relationship.**

### Continuous Quality Improvement in the Eyecare Setting

The popularity of the discipline of total quality management as the basis for continuous quality improvement has become embedded in many successful organizations. Quality in this context is a degree of excellence defined as the ability to meet the customer's needs 100% of the time.[45] The Joint Commission on Accreditation of Health Care Organizations, in 1951, started to ensure the highest possible standards within the industry. Initially, the guidelines of quality assurance addressed the structure, process, and outcomes of the delivery system assessed through provider, facility credentials, and record reviews.[46] In 1992, the commission, which monitors 15,000 health care enterprises, altered the focus of quality to include the disciplines of total quality management and continuous quality improvement (CQI), using the guidelines of W. E. Deming and J. Juran.[47] This new approach to quality assurance accents the need to avoid mistakes rather than surveying what takes place, identifying weaknesses, and making the necessary improvements. CQI programs stress the prime importance of process improvements and a patient-centered approach. The belief is that a practice can best serve patients through a structured approach that reduces system deficiencies and stresses that the ultimate responsibility is to the patient.[48] It is the opinion of some health care analysts that competition in the future will be based primarily on quality.[49]

To ensure the delivery of high-quality service, you need a commitment to performance excellence, a theme that has become popular since appearing in the best-selling book *In Search of Excellence: Lesson's from America's Best-Run Companies* by Peters and Waterman. The authors identify these eight attributes of performance excellence, all of which could be considered standards of performance that ECPs should strive to deliver in their practice:[50]

1. Action bias: Once the decision is made, make sure things are done.
2. Customer relationship: Know their needs and value customer satisfaction.
3. Innovative risk taking: Support entrepreneurship and autonomy.
4. Value human resource contribution: Employee effort produces productivity.
5. Organizational purpose: Understand mission and participation in goal achievement.
6. Core competencies: Emphasize what you do best.
7. Maximum efficiency: Lean staff and flat employee empowered structure.
8. Adaptive style: Be flexible but stay in control.

If you as manager and leader have properly trained your employees about the goals and mission of your practice, the following conversation should never be heard in your office:[51]

Question to staff member: What are your duties?
Staff member's response: I answer the phone, make appointments, and give patients their bills.

Question to staff member: But, isn't it your responsibility to give the best service possible resulting in patient satisfaction? Staff member's response: That's not in my job description.

## Patient Satisfaction Surveys

The importance of measuring patient satisfaction cannot be understated, as many managers of health care practices have recognized. One survey showed that 72.9% of health care providers are developing new methods to evaluate patient satisfaction beyond the commonly used mail questionnaires and surveys.[52] Employee compensation is linked to results, using benchmarks and results from report cards submitted by patients. How is satisfaction actually measured in the health care setting? Another survey revealed that three quarters of practices use mail-in surveys, two thirds perform phone surveys, one twentieth collect patient complaint files, and one twentieth rely on focus groups.[53]

The goal of a patient survey is to ascertain how everyone who matters feels about something in your practice. Obtaining a sample from a portion of your practice that reflects the makeup of your whole practice will allow you to infer what everyone thinks. This sample, or set of patients chosen, should reflect the target population as a whole as best possible to make better decisions. Sample results always are interpreted with confidence levels or error ranges to account for the uncertainty of the process.

A properly administered patient survey can offer valuable insight into how effective your service offering has been. This can be done on completion of the exam as an exit survey, e-mail, or using conventional mail. For the best results, keep the questions of your survey brief, focused, and clear.[54] Using just two questions can be a valuable initial survey. Table 7–1 lists these two questions, based on the encounter points at the patient's visit. By simply asking these two questions about various components of the patient's experience, you can determine which areas to emphasize or exploit and which areas need immediate improvement, as shown in Figure 7–2. Another more detailed satisfaction survey is shown in Table 7–2, which can be used as a marketing tool requesting satisfied patients to refer others. A patient survey of problems experienced

**Table 7-1    Simplified Patient Satisfaction Survey**

---

1. How well did _____ (describe encounter point) meet your expectations?

   Surpassed        Met        Less than

2. How important is _____ (describe same encounter point) to your overall satisfaction?

   Very        Moderately        Not at all

---

|  | **How Well Performed?** | |
|---|---|---|
|  | Poor | Excellent |
| **Very** | Evaluate and revise as a priority | Exploit as primary marketing tactic |
| **Not Very** | Consider discontinuing | If costly, assess if worth continuing |

**How Important?** (row label between Very and Not Very)

**Figure 7-2    Actions to take from a patient survey response.**

directed at improving a provider's office was conducted by Wintersteen Associates on 22,000 patients.[55] The sample responses that follow can be quite enlightening and should be acted on quickly if any arise to prevent problems from occurring:

1. Receptionists need to be more helpful and friendly.
2. Stay on schedule—respect our time.
3. Remember that we are people, not numbers.
4. Justify your fees.
5. Help me understand my insurance benefits.
6. Give assistants more credibility.

### Responding to a Service Delivery Failure

One unfortunate patient response for ECPs is that, according to the consulting firm Granite Rock, 90% of customers who are not satisfied simply stop doing business with a firm rather than offer negative comments beneficial for improvement.[56] "A service failure is essentially a flawed outcome that reflects a breakdown in

**Table 7–2    Detailed Patient Satisfaction Survey**

Our goal is to provide you with the best possible vision care services. To assist us, we would like your comments and feelings regarding the services you have received from our office. Your time and thoughtful consideration in filling out this questionnaire is appreciated. It is not necessary to sign your name unless you wish a personal response. Please enclose this survey in the prepaid envelope or drop it by our office.

Thank You!

|  | *Yes* | *No* |
|---|---|---|
| 1. Did you find it easy to | | |
| Make an appointment at a convenient time? | | |
| Locate our office? | | |
| Find suitable parking? | | |
| Arrange for payment of your bill? | | |
| Please comment: | | |
| 2. Were you satisfied with the | | |
| Services you received? | | |
| Personal attention you received? | | |
| Explanation of your vision problem? | | |
| Explanation of your eyewear options? | | |
| Explanation of the fees charged? | | |
| Promptness and efficiency with which you were cared for? | | |
| Please comment: | | |
| 3. Was our office staff | | |
| Courteous in making your appointment? | | |
| Helpful during your visit to our office? | | |
| Please comment: | | |
| 4. If eyeglasses were ordered for you, | | |
| Were they provided to you at the time promised? | | |
| Was the selection of frames satisfactory? | | |
| Was our fitting and adjustment of your glasses satisfactory? | | |
| Please comment: | | |

*continued*

**Table 7–2** **(Continued)**

|  | Yes | No |
|---|---|---|
| 5. Did any particular person or service make your visit to our office particularly enjoyable or particularly unsatisfactory? Please comment: |  |  |
| 6. What do you feel we could do to make our services more valuable to you and your visits to our office more pleasant? Please comment: |  |  |
| 7. Would you refer a friend to our practice for vision care? |  |  |

Feel free to make additional comments on the back of this form. Thank you for coming to us and referring your friends for our care. We look forward to serving you again!

Respectfully,

---

reliability . . . the cost of unreliable service includes not only the direct expense of redoing the service, but also the indirect penalties associated with the negative publicity generated by displeased customers."[6] An extensive study by Professor Mary Jo Bittner and her colleagues showed that nearly 43% of unsatisfactory service encounters were the direct result of situations handled poorly by employees.[57] Another study by the *Harvard Business Review* reported that two-thirds of customers stop doing business with a firm because they felt unappreciated, neglected, and believed they were treated with indifference.[58]

The attentiveness to detail your office displays during any service recovery episode makes rectifying the situation easier, while influencing a favorable patient outcome. An uninspired recovery effort from a poor service delivery encounter reinforces the patient's attitude that your services are unreliable and produces what Professor Bittner calls a "double deviation" from consumer expectations; the result is a dramatic drop in patient confidence and a migration to the competition.[57]

One final gesture an ECP should offer patients following any service failure is to compensate that patient for the "hassle factor."[59] This is the added cost incurred by the patient created by not performing the promised service correctly the first time. The patient could experience a monetary penalty involved in the expense of returning to your office to rectify the situation or a nonmonetary loss such as the opportunity cost of time spent or stress and frustration created. "An excellent service recovery effort must make amends for the hassle factor . . . do more for the customer than merely reperforming the service . . . make customers feel they gained more than they gave up in going through the recovery process."[15] Actions you could take include giving the patient an added discount, some product for free, or credit their future account. When the patient is directed to the patient lounge (not waiting room) and must wait more than 15 minutes, give a free lottery ticket, as suggested by Vicky Bradford, Ph.D., with a comment like: "Thanks for your patience . . . maybe thanks a million."[60] **An apology alone is not good enough in most cases for the patient inconvenience.**

Empirical studies, such as the Profit Impact of Marketing Strategy (PIMS) database, have documented a positive relationship between perceived quality and higher profit.[61] The study's lead researchers, Buzzel and Gale, show that, in the short term, superior quality enables a business to enjoy higher earnings by being able to charge premium fees while increasing future market share.

Much of the research and literature on evaluating quality is limited to products, but a few conclusions, which follow, can be drawn from the limited number of studies devoted to service delivery:[62]

1. The criteria consumers use to evaluate the quality of a service is much more difficult to understand than how they judge the quality of products.
2. Customers use more than simply the outcome of what they receive from the ECP's practice, they take into account the overall process, including delays or failures.
3. "The only criteria that counts in evaluating service quality are defined by customers. Only customers judge quality; all other judgments are essentially irrelevant. Specifically, service quality perceptions derive from how well a provider performs vis-à-vis customer's expectations about how the provider should perform."[15]

The focus group studies of the classic SERVQUAL research elicited findings that are significant to the ECP.[15] One of these is a definition of customer-perceived service quality that reflects "the extent of discrepancy between customer's expectations and their perceptions." This has evolved into the dominant model of consumer satisfaction with service, referred to previously as the *disconfirmation of expectancy paradigm*. Four parameters were found to influence customer's expectations: what a customer previously might have heard from others, how a customer's specific situation dictates his or her needs, a customer's prior experience, and the communications the customer receives from your practice.

In addition to showing the factors that influence customer expectations, the SERVQUAL study determined four "gaps," or shortcomings, that could influence how a patient derives his or her final perception regarding the quality of your service.[15] First, if the ECP has misconceptions or an erroneous understanding of a patient's expectations, it could lead to unintentional patient dissatisfaction. This could be overcome by the proper use of market research or feedback obtained from patient focus panels and surveys. Second, if the ECP has not adequately defined, erroneously defined, or inadequately conveyed to employees what constitutes high-quality service in that specific setting. This can be accomplished through employee training and monitoring. "When service quality standards are absent or when the standards in place do not reflect customer's expectations . . . quality of service as perceived by customers is likely to suffer."[15] Third, even if the quality of service has been well defined, if there are deficiencies in the way the patient receives the service, the outcome could result in negative patient perceptions. In some instances, especially with very unpleasant patients, it may be advantageous to terminate the relationship.

"To be effective, service standards must not only reflect customer's expectations but also be backed up by adequate and appropriate resources (people systems, technology) . . . employees must be measured and compensated on the basis of performance along those standards."[15] The fourth gap that affects patient perceptions is the discrepancy between what you assert in

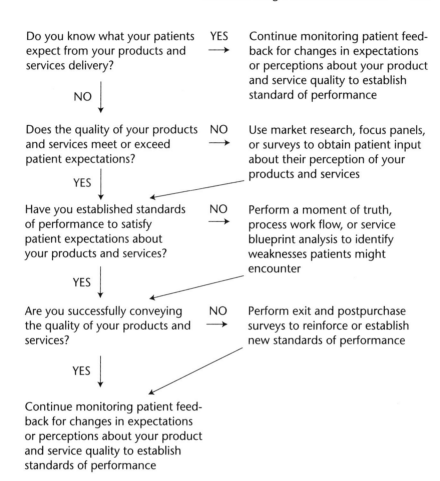

Figure 7–3 Algorithm to establish standards of performance (adapted from Zeithaml V, Parasuraman A, Berry L. *Delivering Quality Service: Balancing Customer Perceptions and Expectations.* New York: Free Press; 1990.

your communications with patients and what you actually deliver. **Coordinating and monitoring your marketing message and educating employees to reinforce that message will make a positive impact on patient perceptions.**

The following is from a poster predominantly displayed at LL Bean, one of the world's leading customer-oriented companies.

While many ECPs may believe the statement to be common sense, one must ask, Is this the same belief held by my employees?

> What is a customer? A customer is the most important person even in this office . . . in person or by mail. A customer is not dependent on us . . . we are dependent on him.
>     A customer is not an interruption of our work . . . he is the purpose of it. We are not doing a favor by serving him . . . he is doing us a favor by giving us the opportunity to do so. A customer is not someone to argue or match wits with. Nobody ever won an argument with a customer. A customer is a person who brings us his wants. It is our job to handle them profitably for him and for ourselves.[63]

Statements of this nature should reflect your commitment to delivering a level of quality service that continually strives to exceed patient expectations and should be conveyed to and exhibited by your entire staff.

The standards of performance you establish for your services ultimately exert a tremendous influence on patient satisfaction. Figure 7–3 describes an algorithm to assist you in establishing desired standards of performance to use as the goal to exhibit in your practice. Once you have established the desired level of staff performance to ensure patient satisfaction, attention can be turned to formulating marketing strategy through planning and analysis of marketing tactics, the topic of the next chapter.

> Exceptional Service . . . No Exceptions
>         —*Roadway Express's promise to customers*

## Action Plan for ECPs

1. Perform sufficient market research to allow you to develop a complete and proper understanding of what your patients expect from your office.
2. Develop service standards for your practice that mirror your patients' expectations and have a favorable impact on the perception your patients make on the quality of your service.
3. Supply the resources, motivate, and direct employees to achieve the desired level of service delivery that will exceed patients' expectations.

4. Assess your communication policies and programs and make sure they accurately convey a message that does not adversely affect the quality of the service your practice delivers. Take all opportunities to enhance their perception of your office and educate patients to the benefits offered.
5. Use either of the sample satisfaction surveys (Tables 7–1 and 7–2) to initiate a patient service improvement program.
6. Train staff members in patient service techniques and offer incentives to enhance service.
7. Anticipate patient expectations, then surpass them.
8. Focus on functional quality dimensions and change your office systems to reduce patient inconveniences.

## Notes

1. Canfield J, Hansen M. *Chicken Soup for the Soul.* Deerfield Beach, FL: Health Communications Inc., 1993.
2. Kanter RM. Transcending business boundaries: 12,000 world managers view change. *Harvard Business Review.* May–June 1991:151–164.
3. Steinhauer J. The undercover shoppers. *New York Times.* February 4, 1998:C1–C2.
4. Sonnenberg F. Service quality: Forethought not afterthought. *Journal of Business Strategy.* September–October 1989:54-57.
5. Massnick F. Customer service can kill you. *Management Review.* March 1997;86(3):33–35.
6. Daniel A. Overcome the barriers to superior customer service. *Journal of Business Strategy.* January–February 1992:18–24.
7. Tschohl J. How to succeed in business by really trying. *Canadian Manager.* Spring 1997;22(1):22–23.
8. Adapted from Donnelly JH, Jr. *Close to the Customer.* Homewood, IL: Irwin; 1992.
9. Christopher M, Payne A, Ballantyne D. *Relationship Marketing.* Oxford: Butterworth–Heinemann; 1996.
10. Berry L, Parasuraman A. *Marketing Services.* New York: Free Press; 1991:5.
11. Berry L. How to sell new services. *American Demographics.* October 1989:42.

12. Spreng R, MacKennzie S, Olshavsky R. A reexamination of the determinants of consumer satisfaction. *Journal of Marketing.* July 1996;60:15–32.
13. Bennett A. Many consumers expect better service—and say they are willing to pay for it. *Wall Street Journal.* November 12, 1990:B1.
14. R. Seger, e-mail, Survey of successful marketing tactics, August 4, 2000.
15. Zeithaml V, Parasuraman A, Berry L. *Delivering Quality Service: Balancing Customer Perceptions and Expectations.* New York: Free Press; 1990.
16. Parasuraman A, Berry L, Zeithaml V. Understanding customer expectations of service. *Sloan Management Review.* Spring 1991:39–48.
17. Trettenero S, Martin G. What a patient says about quality. *Dental Economics.* October 1999:80–81.
18. From Capitol Hill. *Washington Newsletter* [American Society of Ophthalmic Administrators]. May 2000.
19. Ware J. What information do consumers want and how do they use it? *Medical Care.* 1995;33:JS25–JS30.
20. Carson P, Carson K, Roe C. Toward understanding the patient's perception of quality. *Health Care Supervisor.* 1998; 16(3):36–42.
21. Anderson K, Zemke R. Knock your socks off service is reassuring. *American Management Association International.* September 1998:2.
22. Stuller J. Performance and profits. *Training Magazine.* April 1999.
23. Reichheld F, Sasser W. Zero defections: Quality comes to services. *Harvard Business Review.* September–October 1990: 310–307.
24. Sturm A. *The New Rules of Healthcare Marketing.* Chicago: Health Administration Press; 1998.
25. O'Malley JF. *Ultimate Patient Satisfaction.* New York: McGraw-Hill; 1997.
26. Herzlinger R. *Market Driven Health Care.* Reading, MA: Addison-Wesley; 1997.

27. Guillory-Dunbar B. Effects of staff-patient relations training on employees and their feelings about their work. *The Health Care Supervisor*. 1984;13(1):26–30.

28. Thibaut J, Kelly H. *The Social Psychology of Groups*. New York: John Wiley and Sons; 1959:21.

29. Oliver R. A cognitive model of antecedents and consequences of satisfaction decisions. *Journal of Marketing Research* November 1980;17:460–469.

30. Babakus E, Mangold W. Adapting the SERVQUAL scale to hospital settings. *Health Services Research*. 1992;26(6):676–686.

31. Jun M, Peterson R, Zsidisin G. The identification and measurements of quality dimensions in health care. *Health Care Management Review*. 1998;23(4):81–96.

32. Koenig H, Kleinsorge I. Perceptual measures of quality. *Hospital and Health Service Administration*. 1994;39:487–503.

33. Neuwirth Z. An essential understanding of physician-patient communication, part 1. *Journal of Medical Practice Management*. July–August 1999:144–148.

34. Garvin D. Competing on the eight dimensions of quality. *Harvard Business Review*. November–December 1987:101–109.

35. Taylor S. Distinguishing service quality from patient satisfaction in developing health care marketing strategies. *Hospital and Health Services Administration*. Summer 1994;39(2):22–38.

36. Tau H, Cunningham P. Strong opinions held about the tradeoff between choice of providers and cost of care. *Data Bulletin*. Fall 1997:4.

37. Lou Harris Poll 1998. 1,001 Americans describe their health care wish list. *Cost and Quality*. October 1998;4(3):11–14.

38. Study finds doctors don't fully inform patients for decisions. *Boston Globe*. December 22, 1999:A8.

39. Sheridan H, Sheridan G. The right staff. *Management Review*. June 1999:43.

40. Lemmink J, Mattson J. Warmth during non-productive retail encounters. *International Journal of Research in Marketing*. December 1998;5(5):505.

41. Peppers D, Rogers M. When extreme isn't enough. *Sales and Marketing Management*. February 1999;151(2):26.

42. Peltier J, Boyt T, Schibrowsky J. Relationships building. *Marketing Health Services*. Fall 1998:23.
43. D. Lakin, e-mail, Survey of successful marketing tactics, July 27, 2000.
44. Roth K. A tour of the practice through the five senses. *Dental Practice and Finance*. September–October 1999:43–46.
45. Deming WE. *Quality, Productivity and Competitive Position*. Cambridge, MA: MIT Press; 1982.
46. Donabedian A. The quality of care: How can it be assessed? *JAMA*. September 23–30, 1998;260(12):1743–1748.
47. Stoker M. Hospital accreditation standards get tougher. *Orlando Business Journal*. 1993; 43:5.
48. Reeves S, Matney K, Crane V. CQI as an ideal in hospital practice. *The Health Care Supervisor*. 1995;13(4):1–12.
49. Duval C. How will physicians respond. *Medical Care*. 1995; 33:JS31–JS36.
50. Reprinted with permission from Peters T, Waterman R. *In Search of Excellence: Lesson's from America's Best-Run Companies*. New York: Harper and Row; 1982.
51. Modified from a quotation in Shonberger R, Knod E Jr. *Operations Management: Serving the Customer*. Plano, TX, Business Publications; 1988:4.
52. Dunevitz B. Survey: Consumerism drives changes in health care. *Medical Group Management Update*. March 1, 1998:9.
53. Zimmerman D, Zimmerman P, Lund C. *The Healthcare Customer Service Revolution*. New York: McGraw-Hill; 1996.
54. Alreck P, Settle R. The Survey Research Handbook. Boston: Irwin McGraw-Hill; 1995:88–89.
55. Waterman B. The value of value. *Dental Economics*. December 1998:60–64.
56. Customer service: It's what you don't know that's hurting you. *American Management Association International*. July–August 1998:6–7.
57. Bittner M, Booms B, Treault M. The service encounter: Diagnosing favorable and unfavorable incidents. *Journal of Marketing*. January 1990:71–84.
58. Greiner D, Kinni T. *1001 Ways to Keep Customers Coming Back*. Rocklin, CA: Prima Publishing; 1999:128.

59. Firnstahl D. My employees are my service guarantee. *Harvard Business Review.* July–August 1989;4:28–32.
60. Hull B. Patients' moment of truth can occur anywhere in the cycle. *MGM Update.* October 1, 1998:11.
61. Buzzell R, Gale B. *The PIMS Principles—Linking Strategy to Performance.* New York: Free Press; 1987:7.
62. For discussions on evaluating service quality, see Goonros C. *Strategic Management and Marketing in the Service Sector.* Helasingfors: Swedish School of Economics and Business Administration; 1982; Lewis R, Booms B. The marketing aspects of quality. In: Berry L, Shostack L, Upah G, *Emerging Perspectives on Service Marketing.* Chicago: American Marketing Association; 1983:99–107.
63. Peters T, Austin N. *A Passion for Excellence.* New York: Random House; 1985:95.

# CHAPTER 8

# Formulating Your Marketing and Business Strategy

> Our plans miscarry because they have no aim. When a man does not know for what port he is making, then no wind is the right wind.
> —*Seneca, Roman philosopher and senator, first century* B.C.

Strategy is the process of analyzing local marketplace resources, making decisions, and implementing actions to accomplish both your short- and long-term planned objectives. The process is not a one-time event that you put into action but rather a continuous, ongoing sequence of preplanned activities. According to Harry Mintzberg, Ph.D., anyone attempting the strategic planning process should possess the ability to communicate information and have the necessary decision-making capabilities required of all business owners.[1] Although the knowledge to develop strategy is conceptual, to be of value, you must transform the mental images about how you want your practice to develop into a concrete plan of action. Appendix 8–1 offers a self-assessment on the different communication styles you can use with staff to convey and develop marketing and business strategies.

An obstacle that all strategists must reconcile is the paradoxical nature of the "strategic planning" process, which, at times, is inconsistent and contradictory.[2] Strategy development requires a talent for creativity and prediction, both qualitative functions of the brain's right side. This is in contrast to the quantitative nature of planning, which is a left-side brain function that is analytical

193

and requires discipline. According to Richard Cellini, associate vice president of the Strategy Consulting Group, "a left-brain strategy is taking what is and making it better. A right-brain strategy is about taking what is not and making it real."[3]

Factors that affect the development of your strategic plan include the setting of your practice (urban, suburban, or rural), practice entity (solo, partnership, group, or multisite), and what phase your practice presently is in, whether it be starting, expanding, leveling, or declining.

Another significant ingredient is the status of managed care in your local area and how it affects patient volume and access to your office. The phases of managed care in your practice can be thought of as evolving (0–20%), developing (21–40%), in transition (42–60%), penetrating (61–80%), or saturation (81–100%) of your total dollar volume. Other elements include your ability to acquire needed resources and your personal goals. The goals of strategic planning are:[4]

1. Create a unique practice identity different from your competitors.
2. Identify favorable opportunities and potential threats that reduce your risk of uncertainty and develop sustained advantages.
3. Learn how to succeed within a constantly changing business climate.

There are pitfalls that require using caution when confronting staff members with the prospect of developing a strategy. Figure 8–1 is a diagram of these paradoxes. When asserting the control required to initiate strategy, promote discipline to successfully implement each stage of the plan. Control and discipline are compatible; however, to acquire the maximum benefit of staff input, encourage participation by each member, which is the opposite of asserting control. Benefits from participation are realized when each staff member adds individual creativity and, in turn, encourages participation. Take caution not to allow your managerial role of defining discipline stifle your staff's creative potential.

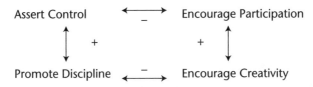

**Figure 8–1    Paradoxical nature of strategist's skills (Vadlamani B. Presentation material given out during lecture in strategic management class of the MBA program, University of Massachusetts, Boston, Summer 1996).**

## Steps in the Strategic Planning Process

The action stages in the strategic planning process follow this basic sequence:[5]

1. Assess current situation.
2. Develop objectives from mission.
3. Collect market research data about competitive environment.
4. Use analytical tools to evaluate the attractiveness of marketplace.
5. Identify key success factors.
6. Formulate a plan.
7. Justify the budget, using a qualitative or quantitative cost-benefit analysis.
8. Implement the plan.
9. Establish controls.
10. Evaluate and revise, if necessary.

Initially, the strategic plan should answer the following general questions; practice-specific questions can be determined once the necessary data have been gathered:[6]

1. Where am I now?
2. Where do I need to go?
3. How will I get there?
4. How will I know when I have arrived?

Begin by developing a profile of your practice that determines what trends within the eyecare industry have led to your current situation. Are future trends favorable to your current model of business strategy? Are you satisfied with the current performance of your eyecare business, or do you need to change strategy and adapt to changes in the marketplace? Answering these questions will give you valuable insight about future avenues you should consider.

## Profit Model Strategies

Two models of profit making are accepted as explaining the choices made when developing strategy: the I/O (industrial organization) model and the resource-based model. The I/O model states that external conditions within the eyecare industry go further to determine the appropriate actions to take than the choices the ECP makes.[7] The ECP's ultimate business performance is a function of the level of competition, established barriers to entry, ability to decrease costs through economies of scale and scope, and ability to offer diversified services and unique products.[8] This model assumes that the resources ECPs use are not exclusive and, therefore, offer no source of advantage for any one ECP. The model implies that first movers have the opportunity to leverage their practice's skills and core competencies to gain advantages.

Conversely, the resource-based model suggests that actions are based on resources and skills within the ECP's capabilities, ultimately limiting the possible number of appropriate actions that can be taken.[9] The ECP's access to specific resources unavailable to the competition forms the basis for realizing marketplace advantages. Only resources that are valuable, rare, costly to imitate, and have no available substitutes can be considered core competencies that become sources of possible advantage over the competition.[10]

In summary, the I/O model assumes all practices in the eyecare industry will use similar learned or obtained strategies, while the resource-based model assumes practices will use different strategies, depending on available resources and capabilities. It seems evident that neither one model exclusively but both in combination explain what occurs in present-day eyecare practice.

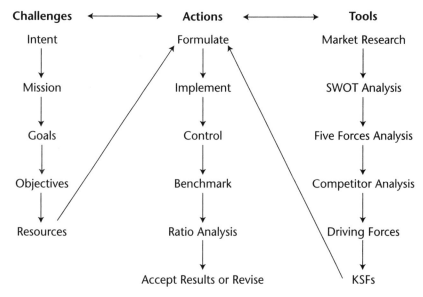

**Figure 8–2   CAT model of strategic planning.**

## The CAT Model

Planning business strategy entails many interrelated business and analytical functions. Figure 8–2 suggests a sequential model we developed for you to follow when formulating your business strategy. The left-hand column, C, lists the challenges you create and must overcome to successfully implement any plan you develop. Creating challenges entails the way you envision your practice evolving and the objectives you have identified. The center section, A, lists the actions you must undertake to actualize your plan. The right-hand column, T, lists the analytical tools to help you assess your marketplace, your competition, and the relative advantages you possess within your drawing area. While at first this may seem an overwhelming task, it is not as demanding as it appears. The preplanning process contributes 80–90% of the finished plan, and once completed, the entire middle column becomes much easier to implement. Therefore, it is important to be as careful as possible about collecting data and making assumptions about your situation.

After developing your practice objectives (found in the left-hand column of the CAT model), proceed to the right-hand column, beginning with an analysis of your external competitive environment. A detailed assessment of your competitive environment includes demographic data, pertinent patient buying behavior, income-expense profitability projections, segmentation strategies, and knowledge of the competition.[3] This is obtained from previous market research analysis used to gather information on both your local marketplace and events or trends in the ophthalmic industry that may influence your decision making. Your external environment provides both resources (customers, materials, information) and patient feedback that will directly affect your profitability.

## Types of Strategic Plans

There are three types of plans you can formulate when making choices. The first deals with your primary strategy addressing the long-term plans you have for your practice, such as diversifying into specialty services and accepting or rejecting specific third party plans. The second type concentrates on the competitive aspects of practice and how to gain advantage over your competitors by adding premium products or expanding coverage. A more-detailed discussion of this topic is found in the upcoming section dealing with generic strategy developed by Michael Porter. The third type of plan focuses on developing the various administrative and operational functions of your practice in areas as marketing, human resource, and finance. This requires you to make adaptive choices to achieve short-term objectives as a response to changes in your local marketplace.

To implement your plan, start by setting policies, developing a budget, and allocating funds. Next, communicate your ideas through personal leadership style and properly motivate your staff to accept your vision. Controls must be established to ensure you set standards to evaluate performance. If you detect any deviations, then corrective measures may be applied.

## Quality as a Strategy

A recent Arthur Andersen/Health Care Forum study showed the prevalence of the following steps in various strategies used by health care managers:

1. Find, train, and retrain high-quality employees.
2. Build network alliances.
3. Invest in patients and employees.
4. Invest in management information services to gain patient buying pattern knowledge.
5. Offer employees economic incentives to enhance customer service.

Yet, with all the talk about the importance of quality improvement, actual measurements between 1996 and 1997 revealed that overall quality improvement measured by the Health Employer Data Information Set (HEDIS version 3.0) increased less than 1%. In fact, in only 1 of the 72 monitored measures was there a noticeable improvement, inclusion of advice to stop smoking increased from 61 to 64% in health plans.

## Five Forces Model of Competitive Analysis

According to Michael Porter of the Harvard Business School, ECPs can gain valuable insight about their relative position by understanding how five industry forces affect their practice:[11]

1. New entrants ease of entry.
2. Presence of substitutes.
3. Leverage of suppliers.
4. Power of customers.
5. Intensity of current rivalry.

If you assess the strength of your competitive position relative to these market forces within the eyecare industry, the resulting analysis should offer you insight to gain advantage over your competition through developing more effective business strategies.

The threat of new entrants directly competing for your patients is a fact of business. Does your area offer only the possibility of lower profit margins due to tremendous competition, the need to continually lower prices, or increasing expenses? Do you need significant capital, specialized knowledge, skills, or brand identity? If potential competitors lack access to these resources, would it be a great obstacle for them to overcome to be successful? If so, these are considered barriers to entry. If there are many barriers to entry or if the barriers are well established, then it is less likely new competitors will enter. As a result, the threat of new entrants is weak. If startup does not have many requirements and barriers to entry are minimal, the threat of new competitors entering your local market becomes stronger. Do you presently have exclusive contracts to provide services, which in effect establishes entry barriers to prevent new eyecare startups in your area? Is your area price sensitive, allowing a low-priced ophthalmic entity to disrupt your market share? Is your location so desirable that a national or regional corporate ophthalmic entity could be tempted to move into your area? What entry barriers can you establish to discourage this from happening? One way is to create a strong brand identity and practice image. **Uniqueness and brands increase loyalty; it is costly for new entrants to overcome patient habits and service to which they are accustomed.**

The second factor consists of substitute products and services. Few, if any, other products or services could be used instead of those in the eyecare industry. A long-term substitute threat may come from technology. If a genetic link is discovered as the cause of refractive errors, it is possible that a future form of gene therapy could eliminate the need for spectacle correction. Refractive surgery has shown significant growth and is entering a more established phase, resulting in slower future expansion and increased consolidation. At the start of 2000, there were 725 refractive surgical centers in this country, a 39% rise over the preceding year.[12] Another possible substitute, physician assistants (PAs) can perform many of the tests typically performed by ECPs. The number of PAs has doubled during the past decade, to slightly over 48,000, and due to the demand, it is likely to increase in the future at a faster pace.[13] At present, the influence of substitutes often can be offset by practice pricing strategies, regulation, and offering high-quality products with innovative features.

The third threat comes from suppliers. What type of business relationship have you established with your vendors? How dependent are you on the ability of your suppliers to deliver the goods you dispense to your patients? Should your suppliers choose to raise wholesale prices, are there alternative sources for you to obtain needed products in order to maintain bottom-line profitability? Does your supplier offer any unique products you can exploit allowing you to differentiate your practice from your competitors? How can you best partner with your supplier to gain competitive advantage? Can you take advantage of co-op advertising or point of purchase promotional materials from your supplier? Your suppliers are a valuable resource to use in differentiating your practice from others. Seek to establish a mutually beneficial and, whenever possible, exclusive relationship with your vendors. Four trends are likely to continue affecting the relationship ECPs have with suppliers:

1. More consolidation, resulting in fewer, larger sources of goods, patients, and materials.
2. More centralization and electronic communication, with incentives for ECPs to do the same.
3. Elimination of sole providers from HMO panels, unless they are part of large groups with which the HMO contracts in order to save costs.[14]
4. Disintermediation, being the direct result of new information technologies: "The advent of certain technologies, such as the Internet, will allow the 'disintermediation' of many processes, eliminating the 'middleman.' This application of technology can dramatically reduce transaction costs, improve consumer convenience and enhance the availability of certain services."[15]

The fourth threat comes from your customers and patients. Do you offer sufficiently unique products and services that patients will continue to value and for which they will be loyal? Are you taking full advantage of consumer trends or fads for maximum profitability? Have you identified the most influential patient groups for services? Do these patients have alternative sources or substitutes that could be used? Can patients easily go elsewhere to buy alternative products or services with no penalty, would they assume little or no switching costs if they chose to abandon your practice? If so, then the threat of the patient is strong. Fortunately, it is evident from the U.S. Bureau of Labor Statistics Eyecare Index that, at present, eyecare offers significant value to patients. The most recent statistics reveal that eyecare consumer costs rose half as much as medical and dental costs for the past 12 years. The past 12-year cumulative consumer eyecare expense rose only 35.3% compared to the Consumer Price Index (inflation rate), which rose 38.7% over the same 12 years.[16] Patient groups are strongest when product and services are undifferentiated and standardized with little switching cost.

The fifth threat is the status of current rivals in your area. Is your area well established due to prior consolidation or is growth still possible due to the fragmented nature of eyecare in your area? What is the market share for your competitors relative to yours? How long have the competitors been established? What has been your competitor's growth trend and why? Does the competition assume an aggressive marketing posture or does it use predatory pricing policies to capture market share? Does it attempt to capture market share through exclusive managed care contracting? What do you anticipate will be the response to each form of strategy you choose to implement? The competition comparison shown in Table 8–1 will help you assess other ECPs in your community while determining potential threats and available marketing opportunities.

A method commonly used to assess competitor strategies is the strategic group map, which highlights and identifies similarities and differences in the type of strategies the major competitors use.[17] Some parameters used to create group maps are

Price
Quality
Image or reputation
Degree and types of service

**Table 8-1  Competition Comparison**

References to obtain information for the profiles include *The Blue Book of Optometrists*, *The Red Book of Ophthalmologists*, *The AOA Directory*, local and county telephone books, sales representatives, the ECP themselves, community members, fellow ECPs, patients, and staff.

| Name and Address | Proximity | Age of ECP | Office Square Footage | Number of Years in Community | Number and Type of Staff | Number of Days in Office | Specialty Offered | Competitive Advantages |
|---|---|---|---|---|---|---|---|---|
|  |  |  |  |  |  |  |  |  |
|  |  |  |  |  |  |  |  |  |
|  |  |  |  |  |  |  |  |  |
|  |  |  |  |  |  |  |  |  |
|  |  |  |  |  |  |  |  |  |
|  |  |  |  |  |  |  |  |  |
|  |  |  |  |  |  |  |  |  |
|  |  |  |  |  |  |  |  |  |
|  |  |  |  |  |  |  |  |  |
|  |  |  |  |  |  |  |  |  |
|  |  |  |  |  |  |  |  |  |
|  |  |  |  |  |  |  |  |  |

Product and service features offered
Location and geographic coverage

The group map in Figure 8–3 shows several different locations providing eyecare that use a variety of different pricing, quality, and image building strategies relative to the type and depth of products and services offered. Compare this to the second group map in Figure 8–4, which shows all the locations offering eyecare using similar strategies.

In summary, if the barriers to entry are strong and well established, the threat of new entry is low or unlikely. However, if the barriers to entry are weak or not secure, then the threat of new entry is high or likely. Many possible substitutes offering eyecare to consumers results in a strong substitute threat to ECPs. If the supplies needed by ECPs to operate the business are scarce, costly, or difficult to obtain from only a few sources, then the supplier threat is high. If patients have no potential loss by changing ECP (no switching cost) and the products or services they require are easily obtained, patient leverage is high, making this a strong threat. A well-established eyecare industry, previously consolidated, offers a strong threat, while fragmentation among existing ECPs offers a weak threat. The challenge for any ECP is to position his or her practice to favorably influence the five industry

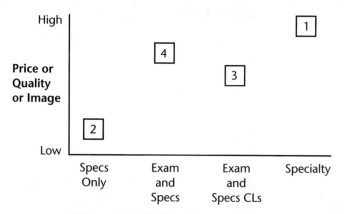

**Figure 8–3   Competitor group map 1, showing various competitors (1–4) use different strategies.**

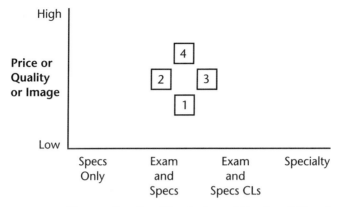

Figure 8–4    Competitor group map 2, showing various competitors (1–4) use similar strategies.

forces that affect eyecare and gain advantage whenever possible to realize better than expected profits.

## Business-Level Strategy

Business-level strategy consists of four options that allow an ECP to provide value to patients by exploiting available resources and capabilities.[18] In the first option, the ECP offers the lowest prices with the goal of becoming the low-cost leader. The second choice finds the ECP offering unique or hard to find products and services at a premium price. These two alternatives can be offered to either a broad range of targets (the general public) or narrow (focus on specific target niches) groups of patients. From these four options the following combined strategies emerge:

1. Broad appeal, low cost.
2. Niche appeal, low cost.
3. Broad appeal, premium cost.
4. Niche appeal, premium cost.

As an example of how the niche/premium strategy led to a successful career, we can heed the words of author-lecturer-practitioner Robert A. Koetting, O.D., F.A.A.O., of St. Louis, who states "if there was ever one factor contributing to my success, it must have been the single goal to identify and excel in a very limited niche market. Everything in my practice and personal life was oriented to providing superior contact lens service for affluent patients, especially presbyopes."[19]

A relatively new fifth alternative is emerging in several industries, including eyecare. The penetration of managed care in several major markets is the spark igniting many ECPs to adopt the strategy of a low-cost, differentiated product, referred to as a *best-cost strategy*, attempting to offer consumers the highest value possible for their dollar. Two strong trends challenge profitability in practice: First, payers and competition force prices down; second, patients demand higher quality. **What is emerging as a necessary strategy is a combination low-cost/differentiation strategy that requires much effort to sustain but, once achieved, creates significant advantage and ultimately patient retention.**

Typically, a low-cost strategy requires focus on internal operations with tight overhead controls and heavy reliance on management information systems to reduce costs. Continual emphasis is placed on reducing expenses and creating strong alliances with networks to gain patients. Relationships with suppliers that offer the most favorable terms are a great advantage. Juxtaposed with the low-cost strategy is a differentiation strategy with an external focus continually enhancing product and service features. Marketing, advertising, and exceptional patient service are vital for this to be successful.

In addition to business-level strategy, decisions must be made concerning competitive-level strategy that reflects the way you compete for and gain market share. Is it through expansion or acquisition of other offices, merging with other providers, diversifying into specialty practice, or first-mover release of new products? If competition is forcing drastic change or affecting revenues, should your mission and objectives remain or change? You must decide about the types of benefits you will emphasize and offer patients.

Core competencies consist of resources and capabilities the ECP practice possesses that affect profitability and the ability to gain market share. Resources include tangible assets, such as the latest technology, equipment, and lenses as well as trained personnel; while intangibles are specialized skills, network alliances, community reputation, and the way you meet patient needs through interaction. The challenge is to assess the adequacy of the resources and skills that become the source of core competencies. Neither resources nor physical assets alone can produce competitive advantages; however, both, in conjunction with practice capabilities, combine to form qualities that make your practice different from the competition. A core competency is "valuable, rare, nonsubstitutable and costly to imitate," and because of these qualities when properly leveraged, it becomes a source of sustained competitive advantage.[9] Value chain capabilities play a role in how the ECP is able to reduce costs when offering a product or service that adds value patients receive and appreciate.[10] What value-creating competencies in the areas of operations, marketing, service, human resources, and technology should you exploit, upgrade, or develop further? You may gain added benefit when patients recognize the added value they receive.

On completion of a thorough internal and external analysis, the answer to the three following questions should be clear:[20]

1. Where in the marketplace should I concentrate my effort?
2. What special services and products do or can I offer current and potential patients?
3. Are my resources and capabilities compatible with the position in the marketplace that I want my eyecare business to occupy?

The answer to the three previous questions will allow the ECP to answer the final and all important question: Is the present strategy I am using to gain sustained competitive advantage for my eyecare business appropriate, or should I change my strategy due to changes in the local marketplace or trends within the ophthalmic industry?

## Driving Forces for Change in Eyecare

In the near future, what factors will influence the way ECPs do business and earn revenue and profits? Your assumptions will identify what you believe to be the driving forces in the eyecare industry; major sources of change are:

1. Diverse interest of the four primary stakeholder group: purchasers, plans, providers, and patients.
2. Changing sources of capital investing in refractive surgery networks, managed care organizations (MCOs), Physician Practice Management Corporations (PPMCs), and corporate chains.
3. Acquisitions, consolidation, and disintegration of practices, corporate entities, HMOs, and networks.
4. Technology advancements in the contact lens industry, refractive surgery, frame and lens materials, exam equipment, and patient communications through the Internet.

The economy, technology, government regulations, and consumer preferences are always changing and exert a large influence on ECP businesses.

Consider the diverse interest of the four primary groups: patients, purchasers, plans, and providers. The priorities patients have are first, value (not lowest cost); second, access to care (ability to contact providers); third, quality of care (often patients are unable to judge); and fourth, quality of service (rapport established, which patients always judge).[21] The American College of Medical Practice Executives believes that the priorities of purchasers (employers), plans, and providers conflict with each other.[22] Purchasers want first, lower prices but improved quality; second, increased buying power through alliances, consolidation, and networks; third, expectations that meet outcomes; and fourth, playing plans against providers. Health plans, on the other hand, want to maintain or raise prices while lowering costs, increase market share, and process information as both an asset for competitive advantage and a commodity to sell for profit while continuing the competition among provider groups.[22] Providers want to maintain incomes, respond to patient needs, and reduce excess capacity that adds to the cost of overhead.

Increased consumer demand and knowledge is another strong force ECPs must deal with in the future. Upward pressure on practice expenses in the face of flat reimbursements due to excess provider capacity will force practices to continually redesign operations for more efficiency. Refractive surgery, expanded therapeutic privileges, and increasing numbers of ophthalmology practices dispensing and opticians refracting all may influence the way ECPs practice. The Internet and demographic changes also will affect the way you practice. **Either your patients will demand that you change or your competitors will force you to change.**

According to a report in *Health Trends,* the "age wave will be the driving force with the greatest influence on the future of American health care and society."[23] With 77 million people born between 1946 and 1964, this segment will become the largest consumer of health care services. Press-Ganey, the country's largest health care satisfaction measuring firm, describes this generation as "consumer-driven, extremely mobile, distrustful of institutions and self-centered."[24]

The challenge for ECPs is to understand the far-reaching influence of the driving forces for change on daily practice and plan appropriately by anticipating the impact of future change and understanding how these changes will influence profitability. Practice trends affecting revenue include your ability to assimilate technology, delegate responsibility, and reduce excess capacity.

You should know the answers to the following questions to buffer any unanticipated events:

1. Where can I develop value-adding activities?
2. What are my most cost-effective activities?
3. What am I doing successfully with specific products and services or segments that I can transfer to other areas?

## Acquisitions and Consolidation

The past decade has produced an inordinately high number of mergers and acquisitions, consolidations, and divestitures in the health care industry. The eyecare sector is no different and certainly not immune to marketplace forces that make the delivery system more efficient and profitable by containing costs. The difference between the value of a single practice and the acquiring entity before and after the merger is called *synergy*. The four variables that form the basis for the increase in mergers and acquisitions are revenues, costs, taxes, and capital requirements.

By changing the four variables that affect cash flow, it is possible to increase the resultant postacquisition synergy, which is a major factor in the increased number of mergers and acquisitions. Synergy can be elevated by increased revenues, decreased costs, lower taxes, or reduced capital expenditures. Revenue increases originate from the larger postmerger practice, which can produce greater revenue than separate practices through marketing efficiencies, more effective promotional efforts, and a better marketing mix. Increased revenue also results from an enhanced position to offer new products and services. A third way is to reduce competition and saturate a geographic area through newly created mergers and cluster marketing. Costs are reduced through greater operating efficiencies and elimination of duplicated expenses through economies of scale and shared overhead, a direct result of mergers. Many eyecare offices do not understand changing marketplace conditions and are unable to abandon old operating strategies. This is overcome by mergers that utilize up-to-date management and information technology systems.

## Key Success Factors

When determining what are the specific key success factors (KSFs) for eyecare, ask, To be successful in the eyecare (ophthalmic) business in this location, what must one do well? Several areas require you to capture certain qualities to exhibit unique, valuable product and service offerings: management skills, communications, operations, marketing, distribution, finance, technology, and organizational capabilities.

The management skills KSFs include being an active listener and delegating not only work but responsibility to your staff for maximum productivity and motivation. According to a recent study by the U.S. General Accounting Office, annual HMO disenrollment is 17%; the reason cited is that nearly half these patients did not like their provider. Patients who have preconceived expectations should receive what is expected to achieve patient satisfaction.

Communication ability is another KSF that should be developed thoroughly. A survey by Relevant Knowledge, Inc., in May 1998, reported that the over age 50 Internet user surfed 19% longer than younger web users. This is obviously an area ripe for development by the eyecare practice because this segment has twice the discretionary income of younger adults and is willing to spend it on health care.[25]

Operations KSFs focus on the optimal utilization of your practice's resources by minimizing excess capacity and inefficiency. This can be accomplished through optimum scheduling effectiveness, striving for a zero no-show rate, and the ability to adhere to budgets and reallocate resources. Training your staff to be as efficient and courteous as possible is essential to a productive business. Continually assimilating the latest management and examining instrumentation technology are also key elements.

Marketing is another KSF that creates a favorable reputation and practice image. Continually identify new ways to deliver your marketing messages such as a website or cooperative and shared marketing. This will give you a lead over the competition and offer the advantages first-movers gain. Using brand identity for uniqueness carries an inherent promise that brand alliance is of greater value or outperforms nonbrand services or products. Plan affiliations or networks like EyeMD create instant added value to the target consumer. One goal of this logo is to differentiate member-providers from others in their respective localities "as the most competent, comprehensive, cost-efficient, convenient and caring providers out there."[26] This could offer competitive advantages should routine eye exams become perceived as a commodity product, because differentiation once this occurs is in many cases neither possible nor profitable.

Distribution KSFs are the various pathways you use to deliver your services to patients and the means by which you obtain patients. Alliances, plans, networks, and employers all assumed major significance in the past decade. But what of the future, will provider unionization or eyecare guilds become a factor? Will out-of-plan options continue to offer perceived value to draw patients? If costs to consumers continue to rise, the number of plans open to providers could decrease due to exclusive agreements offered by health plans. What contingencies do you have in place should this occur? Make sure you can justify the continual need for your services by compiling patient satisfaction surveys.

The finance KSF requires that you develop systems of care that improve productivity and achieve the best and most cost-efficient outcomes with available resources. Access to capital to incorporate the latest technology and ancillary staff for increased efficiency is a necessary and ongoing component of premium quality eyecare delivery.

The technology KSFs include Internet capability for claims processing, EDI, telemedicine, and marketing. You should have a practice website and be communicating with patients electronically for both cost savings and real-time advantage. Most payers are offering incentives to file claims electronically and many will require this in the near future. Patients always are impressed by the latest exam equipment. Make it a high priority to add the latest equipment to your office. Many of these items can be operated by technicians, saving you time and money. The perception the patient receives is that the quality of the exam is enhanced.

The organizational capabilities KSF concerns your ability to adapt third party business regimens by incorporating ongoing continuous quality improvement and retaining an adequately trained and compensated staff. One argument for training employees is that, between 1948 and 1982, 83% of the total growth in the U.S. Gross Domestic Product was attributed to people-related competencies, while only 15% was attributed to investment in capital equipment.[27] Spend as much time and money as you can on training your employees, it is one of the best investments you can make. Employees are a key source of gaining competitive advantage for every business.

On completion of an analysis of the practice's external marketplace, you can, with confidence, evaluate which opportunities seem attractive. In addition, you should recognize any trends threatening your practice's stability and profitability. With this information, you have a better understanding of what is required to gain sustained competitive advantage and differentiate your practice from your local competitors. Appendix 8–2 shows how to develop a marketing plan to add a specialty service. After you complete this, Appendix 8–3 offers possible solutions. Once you have selected specific opportunities to pursue, proper implementation and control (the topic of Chapter 9) are necessary functions to ensure the success of your marketing endeavors.

## Action Plan for ECPs

1. Review all the preliminary data and material you have gathered in the planning stage. Have you overlooked any steps?
2. Perform a five forces analysis (see p. 199) to assess your position relative to the forces that influence your success.
3. Complete the Competition Comparison (Table 8–1) to assess other ECPs in your community. Assess your position relative to the competition.
4. Decide what type of business-level strategy you want to use and how broad or narrow a focus you want to take reaching your target groups.
5. Determine if any forces for change offer you some opportunity to take advantage of or a potential threat you must anticipate and take a specialized course of action.
6. Identify the KSFs you must either possess or obtain for you to achieve your marketing program and business goals.
7. Complete Identifying Your Business Communication Style (Appendix 8–1) prior to initiating any marketing strategy with your staff.
8. Complete the Specialty Service Marketing Program (Appendix 8–2) for a specialty service or new product you want to offer.

# Identifying Your Business Communication Style[28]

Place a 4 next to the response you would most likely to make, a 3 next to the response you would make second, a 2 next to the response you would make third, and a 1 next to the response you would least likely make.

1. A staff member failed to track the monthly marketing expense report on time.
   ____ a. Tell that person to complete the report immediately.
   ____ b. Ignore it since the report is not really important to the profit of the practice.
   ____ c. Discuss the benefit to your practice of filing the report on time.
   ____ d. Discuss the reasons why the report was not completed, clarify the personal benefit to the staff person of completing the report while stressing the importance that it be completed as soon as possible.

2. You have asked a staff member to develop a marketing plan for your eyecare practice based on the goals and objectives outlined in your office policy manual.
   ____ a. Evaluate what the member already has done and recommend that he or she continue.
   ____ b. Give the member a training manual on developing a marketing plan for an eyecare practice.
   ____ c. Encourage and praise the member's efforts up to this point.
   ____ d. Meet with the member and describe your specific goals and jointly determine what steps should be taken next.

3. A consultant told you that you need to implement a new business strategy for your eyecare business due to decreased productivity.

_____ a. Review everyone's job description and tell everyone how his or her duties fit into the new strategic plan.

_____ b. Call a short meeting to inform the entire staff about the consultant's plan.

_____ c. Informally discuss with members of your staff the benefits of developing new strategy.

_____ d. Meet with each staff member and jointly determine ways of implementing specific suggestions.

4. You budgeted money to send one staff member to attend a course in business principles at the local community college.

_____ a. Pick the person you think would benefit most, and tell this individual to attend.

_____ b. Ask the staff who would like to attend, and if there is more than one, let the staff choose who you will send.

_____ c. Determine who could benefit the most by attending, and discuss the matter with that staff member before you make a choice.

_____ d. Call a meeting to discuss the benefits of attending with the entire staff, and jointly determine who would benefit the most by attending.

5. During a recent meeting, your staff told you that you are the reason for the poor productivity in the office and they are all working their maximum in order to receive the large bonus you promised based on end-of-year revenues.

_____ a. Tell the staff you absolutely disagree and mention some examples to support your claim.

_____ b. Don't say anything. They obviously don't know what they're talking about.

_____ c. Tell them that you are as interested in increasing productivity as they are. Ask them to tell you what they have been doing to handle the problems.

_____ d. Ask the staff why they believe you are the problem, and together try to identify specific steps that can be taken to deal with the problem.

*Instructions.* Copy your responses onto the following answer sheet by matching the letter of each answer. For example, in situation 1, if you placed 3 next to the choice a, 2 next to choice b, 4 next to choice c, and 1 next to choice d, enter across row 1 the numbers 3, 2, 4, 1, respectively. Use this same approach to enter your response for the remaining situations.

|  | a | b | c | d |
|---|---|---|---|---|
| Situation 1 | ____ | ____ | ____ | ____ |
| Situation 2 | ____ | ____ | ____ | ____ |
| Situation 3 | ____ | ____ | ____ | ____ |
| Situation 4 | ____ | ____ | ____ | ____ |
| Situation 5 | ____ | ____ | ____ | ____ |
| Total | ____ | ____ | ____ | ____ |

*Scoring and explanation.* The higher the total in a column, the more it indicates your leaning toward that style. Column a represents an autocratic (aggressive) communication style. Column b represents a laissez-faire style (avoidance or what will be, will be) style. Column c represents a paternalistic (compromising style), and Column d represents a participative (collaborative) communication style. While all four styles are used with subordinates, the participative style usually is considered the most effective.

# Sample Specialty Service Marketing Program

Using the information from previous chapters on the various components that make up a marketing program, complete the following to add a new pediatric vision training specialty. After completing this portion, turn to Appendix 8–3 for examples of solutions.

1. The purpose of my marketing is to _____
2. I will achieve this purpose by focusing on the following benefits offered: _____
3. The target groups are _____
4. The marketing techniques I will use are _____
5. My image and brand identity will be _____
6. The budget I will allocate for this is _____

Take your answers to the above questions and complete the following detailed marketing program.

1. Mission:
   _____
   _____

2. Objectives (use the SMART acronym):
   _____
   _____

3. Market research required:
   _____
   _____

4. SWOT:
   _____
   _____

5. Service life cycle message:

   _____

   _____

6. Segments and target groups:

   _____

   _____

7. Marketing mix (how will you use the four *P*s):
   Place:

   _____

   _____

   Promotion:

   _____

   _____

   Product:

   _____

   _____

   Price:

   _____

   _____

8. Assess effectiveness:

   _____

   _____

9. Budget:

   _____

   _____

# Possible Solutions for Developing a Pediatric Vision Training Marketing Program

1. *Mission.* To develop a pediatric vision care specialty constituting 20% of my practice revenue within 2 years.
2. *Objectives.* Within 1 year to have completed 25 initial evaluations and enrolled 20 school-age children in a vision training (VT) program. By the third year to have two initial new evaluations per week, enroll 40 children, and employ one full-time binocular vision training technician.
3. *Market research.* Obtain information on the percentage of families with school-age children and per capita income greater than $50,000 within radii of 1, 3, 5, and 10 miles from my office.
4. *SWOT.*
   *Strength.* Well-established primary care practice, VT residency.
   *Weakness.* Inadequate time to make personal presentations as marketing tactic.
   *Opportunity.* No VT specialist within 20 miles.
   *Threat.* Local group medical practice could hire an independent orthoptist.
5. *Life cycle message.* Introductory phase awareness and information.
6. *Segments and target groups.*
   Parents of school-age children
   Teachers
   School nurses
   Pediatricians
   Learning development institutes
   Child psychologists
   School-age children

7. *Marketing mix choices.*

   Public relations appearances, personal presentations, publicity, direct mail, and giveaways.

   *Place.* Point-of-sale in-office materials and announcements, build a children's area in patient lounge, school visits, mailed print media, news media.

   *Promotion.* Discuss the benefit of VT through educational presentations one on one to school nurses, teachers, child psychologists, and learning development institutes after a direct mail to previously identified recipients. Group presentations to parent organizations. In-class posters and teacher manuals including lesson plans.[29] Direct mail newsletter to select current patients most likely to use or recommend services. Perform vision screenings and donate books on eye health to schools. Submit consumer information articles to local newspaper.

   *Product.* Message will emphasize the benefits gained through VT.

   *Price.* Introductory package prices and one free initial consultation until established.

8. Budget 10% of projected annual gross revenue for this service.

## Notes

1. Mintzberg H. Crafting strtategy. *Harvard Business Review.* July–August 1987;65(4):66–77.
2. Mintzberg H. *The Rise and Fall of Strategic Planning.* New York: Free Press; 1994:5.
3. Morrall K. Piecing together a strategic plan. *Bank Marketing.* September 1996;28(9):26–34.
4. Coile R. Strategic planning for the millennium. *Russ Coile's Health Trends.* December 1997;10(2):3.
5. Adapted from Freitag A. PR planning primer. *Public Relations Quarterly.* Spring 1998:14–17.
6. Freitag A. PR planning primer. *Public Relations Quarterly.* Spring 1998:14–17.
7. Schendel D. Introduction to competitive organizational behavior. *Strategic Management Journal.* Winter 1994:2.
8. Seth A, Thomas H. Theories of the firm. *Journal of Management Studies.* 1994;31:165–191.
9. Barney J. Firm resources and sustained competitive advantage. *Journal of Management.* 1991;17:99–120.
10. Barney J. Looking inside for competitive advantage. *Academy of Management Executive.* 9(4):56. Lado A, Boyd N, Wright P. A competency based model of sustainable competitive advantage. *Journal of Management.* 1992;18:77–91.
11. Adapted with permission from Porter M. *Competitive Strategy.* New York: Free Press, 1980.
12. Moretti M. Large corporations dominate the LVC food chain. *EyeWorld.* December 1999:16.
13. Lenkiewicz A. PAs lend expertise as well as efficiency to your practice. *EyeWorld.* September 1999:70.
14. HMOs dumping doctors who don't join big groups. *The Lowell Sun.* December 24, 1999:3.
15. Glaser J, Hsu L. *The Strategic Application of Information Technology in Healthcare Organizations.* New York: McGraw-Hill; 1999.
16. Eyewear, care costs slightly outpaced inflation in 1999. *AOA News.* March 6, 2000; data from the Bureau of Labor Statistics.

17. Peteraf M, Shanley M. Getting to know you: A theory of strategic group identity. *Strategic Management Journal.* 1997; 18:165–186.
18. Porter M. *Competitive Advantage: Creating and Sustaining Superior Performance.* New York: Free Press; 1985.
19. R. A. Koetting, e-mail sent July 26, 2000.
20. Corporate strategy: a manager's guide. *Harvard Management Update.* January 2000;5(1):1–4.
21. According to a survey by the Center for Research in Ambulatory Health Care Administration (CRAHCA).
22. Davis K. Major system dynamics drive health care. *Medical Group Management Update.* July 1, 1998:6.
23. *Russ Coiles Health Trends.* July 1998;10(7).
24. Regrut B. The Boomer consumers and health care. Press-Ganey [South Bend, IN] on-line report. 1998:1–10.
25. Dychtwald K. *Age Wave: The Challenges and Opportunities of an Aging America.* Los Angeles: J. P. Tarcher; 1998.
26. Dunleavy B. The EyeMDs have it. *Vision Monday.* December 14, 1998:6.
27. Nussbaum B. Needed: human capital. *Business Week.* September 1988:100.
28. Modified from Gibson JW, Hodgetts RM. *Business Communication: Skills and Strategies.* New York: Harper & Row; 1990: 24–25.
29. ABCs of Eyecare Program, Better Vision Institute, Washington, DC, 1996.

# CHAPTER 9

# Implementing and Controlling Your Plan

"I can't do it," never accomplished anything. "I will try," has performed wonders.

—*G. P. Burnham*

Strategy implementation involves information systems utilization of external data and market research. Once your plan is developed, the necessary changes must be accepted as your new practice identity, reflecting the values, capabilities, and tactics that will determine the degree of success. Precautions must be taken against any resistance by staff members to changes in established practice protocols. You should predict staff opposition by obtaining feedback. Consider assigning various individuals responsibility for portions of the implementation process. The five-step process shown in Table 9–1 can guide you throughout the implementation of your plan.

When evaluating and refining your plan, answer the following questions:

1. Are my goals and objectives properly addressed?
2. Are the requirements (key success factors) for success sufficiently identified?

**Table 9–1    Strategy Implementation**

---

Step 1. Understand all factors required to successfully achieve your plan.

Step 2. Describe what you want to achieve, who is involved, their roles, and the resources required.

Step 3. Understand the current situation and how you want it to change

Step 4. Create a sequential list of the events required to achieve your objectives.

Step 5. Once you have assessed your readiness and ability to take action, initiate your plan.

---

Modified from Stock B. Leading small-scale change. *Training and Development*. February 1993; 47(2):45–50.

3. Have all essential business systems and operations procedures been properly assessed for functional adequacy?
4. Have the desired objectives and required resources been benchmarked to the ideal outcome?

Typically, you will find that "when a problem is well-formulated, the problem is half solved."[1] This is similar to taking a good case history and applies to the implementation of a strategic plan. If you are not achieving results you want, look for problems in the following areas: poor management decisions, poor product or service, inadequate resources, lack of core capabilities, insufficient capital, or weak marketing.

Symptoms of problems such as employee turnover or downward trends in revenue and profits should be addressed as well. How has your choice of short- and long-term strategies enhanced your ability to remediate problems you may encounter?

To properly monitor the level of your strategy's realized accomplishment, you must establish standards of performance and benchmarks of your progress. This is done by tracking and comparing your results in a given time period to prior results and other practices, when this information is available. Evaluate actual performance and detect departures from predetermined desired results. By detecting deviations from what you anticipate early, you have the opportunity to apply corrective measures to avoid an unsuccessful turnout.

## Benchmarking

Benchmarking dates back to Alexander the Great, who after comparing the advantages his enemies enjoyed, would revise his strategy and tactics. In 1979, Xerox Corporation was the first modern-day company to apply concepts of benchmarking to its business operations, after its market share fell to 35% from 80% due to intense competition from expanding overseas companies. Keep in mind that "benchmarking is not imitation or copying, it is an opportunity to learn and assimilate new data."[2] ECP offices handle a mix of clinical, managerial, and operational procedures with a very small likelihood of making all possible processes "the best." However, exert caution: Benchmarking often detects deficient performance and this could become an unattainable barrier better left undetected. Applying too stringent or idealistic a level of performance to achieve may produce unintentional practice problems.

The term *benchmarking*, as it applies to the eyecare setting, can take on several meanings, using a variety of methods to achieve many different outcomes that offer direction to improve practice performance. "Simply stated, benchmarking is the sharing of performance information to identify the operational and clinical practices that lead to the best outcome."[3] By using realistic benchmarks, improvements can be made in patient satisfaction, employee morale, and practice financial performance.

Benchmarking has been described as a "comparison process that becomes a hunt for new opportunities and improvements for healthcare organizations."[2] It can be applied to various practice areas, including finance, operations, patient service and satisfaction, human resource management, and marketing. Practice finance and operations benchmarks by specialties are available from The National Association of Healthcare Consultants, and the Society of Medical-Dental Consultants. An example for medical eyecare practices from a 1999 report showed that the ratio of full-time employees to provider was 5.63 for dispensing practices and 4.56 for nondispensing practices. Also, in both types of practice, staff wages constitute 20.7% of total revenue.[4]

Benchmarks offer a way to objectively measure staff productivity and the quality of service your practice delivers. Signals that indicate you should consider benchmarking include negative patient or employee feedback, negative remarks on patient surveys, poor financial performance, and increased levels of personal frustration with the way your practice is going.[5]

Benchmarking can be applied to achieving an objective as simple as improving a single practice expense to the complex issue of attaining improved performance levels for a quality assurance program. Benchmarking is "the strategy which results in the customization of projects to suit an organization's needs and requires data sharing and networking to create positive outcomes."[6] According to the Medical Group Management Association (MGMA), it is "the use of external data to compare internal processes. In health care, benchmarking is used to compare costs and productivity and to detect industry trends."[7] As an example, a MGMA survey found that most outpatient health care offices average approximately four full-time staff members for every provider.[8] But in an eyecare office, depending on services offered, automation used, and staff efficiency, this number easily could range from three to five.

The benchmarking process starts with the collection of operating data associated with measurements of performance from available practices and resources. Next, the best performance indicators are identified; finally, the ECP adapts the practices that produce the best results for his or her setting with the goal of improving performance. Do not confuse quality assurance (QA) with benchmarking. QA identifies results or practices that are inferior to an established minimum level of acceptability. Once identified, the behavior deemed unacceptable is either eliminated or remediated. In traditional QA programs, the focus is strictly on isolating and correcting below standard performance. Benchmarking, however, takes into account the entire practice and attempts to achieve the best possible operational performance. It "helps measure where we are, and helps us understand where we need to go."[5]

To obtain insight for a practice, five primary benchmark comparisons may be used.[3] The first is an internal focus on the components of ongoing practice operations. The second is obtained by surveying the competition. The third is functional in nature, making comparisons to the performance exhibited by the most successful practices in the industry. The fourth is a comparison to other ECP practices in the same network. The fifth chosen benchmark is a comparison of your results to the best of class in other industries. For example, this last benchmark might involve obtaining data on customer service delivered by Southwest Airlines, a company where the employees are known to pride themselves on obtaining the highest possible customer satisfaction ratings. Benchmarking is intended to help assess how and where to improve performance or patient satisfaction, cut costs, or allocate resources and the value of choosing one practice pattern over another.

Common errors in benchmarking include initiating data collection as a one-time event. **Benchmarking is an ongoing process that requires the participation of your entire office, not just for data collection but to implement change once those areas in need are identified.** Another downfall occurs when a practice tries to directly incorporate what others are doing. Make sure your goals are explicit and accepted by all involved staff members. Avoid fixing isolated parts of systems. Understand the entire sequence of events involved in benchmarking targets to ensure that no one element of any process is left unaligned.[9]

## Best Practices

Benchmarking is most successful when the "best practices" are adapted to the needs and peculiarities of your practice by taking into account your specific situation. Make sure the system of measurement is the same for your practice as to the practices against which you benchmark, or else the conclusions you draw will be of little value. Areas in eyecare where best practices data can be applied are to improve patient outcomes and administrative efficiency, to reduce operating cost, and to use as support when contracting with managed care organizations.[10]

Caution is required when using the Internet as a source of data for comparison. The quantity of information could become a burden without the proper use of advanced search engines. Advice on using search engines to find best practice information is found on the website of Future Healthcare's WebCenter for Clinical Informatics (www.futurehealthcare.com). The quality of the information to be found on the Internet must be evaluated carefully as to its worthiness. This was clarified by an editorial in a recent issue of the *Journal of the American Medical Association*, which stated, "At first glance, science and snake oil may not always look all that different on the Net."[11] It is recommended that all best practice information you use be supported by a disclosure that describes the evidence used and how the conclusions were drawn.[12]

If you decide to begin a benchmarking program, consider making comparisons to the best performance of companies in other industries, not only eyecare. For example, patients' willingness to wait is greatly influenced by their experiences in other places, such as the speed of service typical of most fast food restaurants or what computer technology offers. They will make this comparison when they are in the patient lounge waiting in your office.

It is generally accepted that benchmarking is performed to ensure the highest levels of patient satisfaction as the primary goal. However, at times, it can be difficult to determine the parameters that create a patient's perceived level of satisfaction. In 1994, the American Customer Satisfaction Index was started to assist the process of quantifying satisfaction.[13] This index is the result of an alliance between the Business School at the University of Michigan, the American Society for Quality, and Arthur Andersen. "It is the only uniform, cross industry measure of consumer's perception of goods and services in the United States and the first to link customer satisfaction to bottom-line, financial results."[8] Sources of comparative data may be found at professional conventions, by obtaining data tabulated by sales reps, on the Internet, obtained through surveys performed by the national professional organizations, and by surveying your peers. An example of benchmarking, shown in Table 9–2, uses numeric data to make operational comparisons in a fee-for-service medical practice. This data can be found on the Medical Group Management Association website (www.mgma.com).

Another type of benchmarking that can be performed involves quality as the measured parameter, using feedback from

**Table 9-2    Selected 1997 Median Operating Costs per Full-time Equivalent Provider**

| | |
|---|---|
| Total support staff cost | $124,365 |
| Total support staff benefits | $23,612 |
| Information services | $6,733 |
| Building and occupancy | $26,049 |
| Furniture and equipment | $6,626 |
| Administrative supplies and services | $7,004 |
| Promotion and marketing | $2,097 |
| Total operating costs | $239,695 |

Reprinted with permission from Medical Group Management Association cost survey, 1998.

patient surveys. A sample of questions that the ECP can ask patients is shown in Table 9–3. Specific business practices that contribute to the success of better performing offices have been identified, including establishing a mission, goals, objectives, operating policies, and procedures that focus on maximizing efficiencies.[14] Incentives are used for hard work, effort, cost control, and efficiency. Investments are made into quality management with continual enhancements in practice information systems to improve quality and decrease costs.

**Table 9-3    Service Quality Questions**

How thorough was the exam?

Did the staff seem to express adequate concern for your problems?

Do you feel you were given adequate time to address your problem?

Do you believe you were given adequate advice to resolve your problem?

Did you have adequate access to this office?

Was the waiting time acceptable?

What was your overall satisfaction with this office?

## Financial Ratio Analysis

Comparing the performance of specific areas of an ECP's operations to established industry norms offers a method of assessing overall performance. One of the most commonly used approaches involves financial ratio analysis. One often used ratio that indicates the solvency or liquidity of a business is the *current ratio* calculated by dividing *current liabilities* into *current assets*. The median current ratio for optometric offices under one million dollars in annual revenue is 1.3 times, and the range for all optometric practices is 0.4–2.3.[15] Books containing industry norms of financial ratios can be found in the reference section of most university or larger public libraries. The most popular books on this subject are *Annual Statement Studies* by Robert Morris Associates, *Industry Norms and Key Business Ratios* by Dun & Bradstreet, and *Almanac of Business and Industrial Financial Ratios* by Leo Troy. There are four major types of financial ratios: profitability, liquidity, activity, and leverage.

An understanding of financial documents and calculations is necessary to gain the maximum benefit from the application of financial ratio analysis. The ECP with limited financial experience should consult an accountant and use a basic finance text. Profitability or performance ratios that the ECP would find useful include three profit margins—gross, operating, and net—as well as return on assets and equity. Profitability or performance ratios indicate how successful you are earning revenue and profits given the practice's resources and assets. Liquidity ratios include both the current and quick ratios, which measures the ability of the practice to meet current debt obligations. Activity or operating ratios indicate how effective and efficient practice assets are being utilized. These include four turnover ratios (inventory, fixed assets, total assets, and accounts receivable) as well as average collection period. Finally, leverage ratios that reveal the extent borrowed funds are used to finance practice operations include ratios of debt to asset, debt to equity, and long-term debt to equity.

Financial accounting methods can accurately track, measure, and monitor operating costs per service. It is important to identify and develop user-friendly systems that promote efficient service delivery for all the various "customers" of the practice (patients, employers, insurers, referral sources). As an example, one authoritative source, Essilor Labs of America, has identified the "capture rate" benchmark in the average ophthalmology dispensary as 45–55% with a range of 28–80%.[16] Another ratio that can be quite helpful to benchmark is the dispensary's frame inventory turnover. This is simply the dollar volume of optical sales divided by the average annual wholesale cost of the frame inventory on hand. To determine this ratio, first add the dollar amount of the year's beginning and ending optical frame inventory and divide by 2. This amount is the average annual wholesale cost of the frame inventory. Divide this amount into the annual gross revenue for frame sales. The resultant figure is the inventory ratio. If gross frame sales are $200,000 and average frame inventory is $25,000, the inventory turnover ratio is 8 times. The normal range for the frame inventory turnover in optical dispensaries is between 6 and 8 times in a year.[16]

Analyzing the implication of a financial ratio can offer insight for strategic planning of your eyecare business. A low inventory turnover ratio implies that you are not adequately utilizing your assets, in this case your inventory, to the fullest possible extent. This may signal that either more training and monitoring is required in optical sales, or, alternatively, you do not need to carry such a large frame inventory. On the other hand, a high ratio may indicate that your present frame inventory is not sufficient to service the current demand signaling the need to carry a larger inventory. Table 9–4 lists some of the indicators that can be used to identify differences between "typical" practices and "better performing" practices.

In the future, consider adding other variables of a nonfinancial nature to benchmarking. Don't simply focus your attention on comparisons of internal measurements of practice expenses. Consider external measurements, which include market share, patient satisfaction, patient retention, employee satisfaction, alliances, and outcomes. Use the following as possible benchmarks to establish your standards of performance:

1. Number of exams per hour.
2. Number of patients per day.

**Table 9–4    Indicators Used to Differentiate Better Performing Practices**

---

I. Practice Operating Efficiency and Profit
   1. Gross and net revenue per provider.
   2. Operating cost per provider.
   3. Operating cost as a percentage of gross revenue.
   4. Net revenue as a percentage of gross revenue.
   5. Operating costs per service.

II. Staff Efficiency
   1. Support staff costs per provider.
   2. Nonsupport staff costs per provider.
   3. Costs per square foot.

---

Modified from Medical Group Management Association. *Performance and Practices of Successful Medical Groups: 1998. Report Based on 1997 Data.* Englewood, CO: Medical Group Management Association; December 1998.

3. The percentage capture rate for product sales from your exams.
4. The percent of patients with service complaints.
5. Changes in capacity utilization and excess capacity.

Ultimately, some form of activity-based cost analysis using Health Care Finance Administration's (HCFA) relative value unit scale may be the most accurate method of quantifying practice expense analysis.

## Benefits Gained by Planning for the Future

Distance planning is difficult in the eyecare industry, with a number of variables confronting ECPs. Planning beyond 3 years presents hazards and, in most cases, is ill-advised. Changes in industry structure may offer insight into directions worth pursuing. Consider the following questions when deciding on future avenues to take:

1. What will the structure of the eyecare industry be in 10 years?
2. What skills, capabilities, and resources will be required to be successful as an ECP?

3. What are probable sources of competitive advantage for ECPs?
4. What entities play the major roles in challenging the accepted paradigms and developing new and better ways to deliver eyecare?
5. What will be the driving forces for change and what entities will assume positions of leadership in the eyecare industry?

In the future, the eyecare profession might benefit by monitoring specific marketplace variables that are critical to a better understanding of forces influential to business performance. Developing and monitoring a new discipline (optonomics, ophthalmonomics, or oculonomics) that measures the impact these variables have might be a first step. Data collected could focus on changes in the eyecare delivery system, regulatory mandates, clinically required protocols, and consumer preferences. Outcomes of the study could identify the most favorable methods ECPs have used to adapt to marketplace change.

On completion of your strategic planning process, you should have formed concrete ideas to follow in areas of practice development, revenue enhancement, or patient satisfaction by:

1. Articulating the future vision of your practice.
2. Providing direction consistent with your long-term objectives.
3. Offering a framework for implementation and resource allocation.
4. Directing financial, managerial, and human resource decision making.
5. Describing benchmarks of performance and achievement.

Although the complete process of developing marketing strategy may seem an arduous task, many rewards come from a systematic, disciplined, well-formulated approach. The wisdom of 25 centuries ago still offers insight today for those attempting to develop marketing strategy for their business: "Those who understand strategy move without delusion and progress without tiring. Know nature and know the situation."[17]

## Action Plan for ECPs

1. Identify the areas of your practice you want to improve by using benchmarks to compare your performance to that of others.
2. Develop a meaningful system for measuring results, either qualitatively through patient and staff feedback or quantitatively using numerical data that your office collects.
3. Determine methods to implement change for the areas that your benchmarking indicates need improvement.
4. Consider forming a small discussion group of colleagues to compare findings.
5. Begin to monitor changes in a few key financial parameters by using financial ratio analysis to assist you in recognizing areas that may require closer attention.

## Notes

1. Murdick R. *Business Research: Concepts and Practice.* Scranton, PA: International Textbook Company; 1987.
2. Paz H, Livingston J. Using benchmarking system to improve patient care and assist in technology assessment. *Physician Executive.* March 1996;22(3):10–12.
3. Czarnecki M. Benchmarking strategies for healthcare management. *Hospital Cost Management Accounting.* 1996;7(10):8.
4. Compare your staffing costs with national averages. *Medical Office Staff Management Strategies.* 1999.
5. Schecter K. Benchmarking requires objective staff involvement. *American Medical News.* January 11, 1999;42(12):22.
6. Kreider C, Walsh B. Benchmarking for a competitive edge. *Medical Laboratory Observer.* September 1997;29(9):26–27.
7. Adams T. Benchmarking becoming vital for physician success. *American Medical News.* March 10, 1997;40(10):27.
8. Redling B. Benchmarks provide starting points for projecting staff needs. *MGM Update.* December 1, 1997:4.
9. Gelinas M, James R. Is your benchmarking missing the mark? *Healthcare Benchmarks.* June 1999;6(6):68–70.

10. Kibbe DC, Smith PP, La Vallee R, et al. A guide to finding and evaluating best practices health care information on the Internet: the truth is out there? *Journal of Quality Improvement.* December 1997;23(12):678–689.
11. Silberg WM, Lundberg GD, Musacchio RA. Assessing, controlling, and assuring medical information on the Internet. *JAMA.* 1997;277(15):1244–1245.
12. Hayward RS, Wilson MC, Tunis SR, et al. How to use clinical practice guidelines: Are the recommendations valid? *JAMA.* 1995;274(7):570–574.
13. Clarke B, Sucher T. Benchmarking for the competitive marketplace. *Journal of Ambulatory Care Management.* July 1999; 22(3):72–78.
14. Shryver D. Question: What is a better-performing practice? *Medical Group Management Journal.* July–August 1999; 46(4): 6–8.
15. Robert Morris Associates Annual Statement Studies, 1999–2000. Chicago, IL, p. 1177.
16. Gardner B. Benchmarking the optical dispensary. *Administrative Eyecare.* Fall 2000;9(4):23–26.
17. Sun Tzu, *The Art of Strategy*, translated by Wing RL. New York: Doubleday; 1988.

# CHAPTER 10

# New Marketing Technology

## Internet Marketing

E-commerce is dramatically changing the way many industries do business. The impact of this trend on the patients of an eyecare business remains to be seen. Any eyecare business that utilizes the Internet must identify and reach target segments offering the most profit potential by creating perceived value that serves patients' needs. "How well the Web works for a company depends on old-fashioned smarts and elbow grease. It isn't glamorous at all. The difference between Web success and Web failure often hinges on how carefully people sift through the details and fine-tune niggling plans."[1]

Cyberspace offers the ECP new marketing opportunities not available just five years ago. (For your information, the term *cyberspace* was coined by William Gibson in the 1984 novel *Necromancer*.) User traffic on the Internet doubles every four months and Internet content grows by 300,000 pages per week.[2] This indicates the likelihood that more of your existing and potential patients are using this tool as a medium to gain access to information and purchase products, often at the expense of more traditional media used by ECPs. The latest statistics reveal a 13% drop in television viewing, an 8% decrease in weekly magazine readers, and 5% loss in daily newspaper use.[3] The implication is this: a huge subculture of consumers that use the Internet for current events and shopping is emerging. Another estimate claims that there already are 15,000 health-related websites.[4] ECPs that take a more progressive marketing approach will be the first to

**Table 10–1  Growth of Various Communications Media**

| Type | Years |
|------|-------|
| Radio | 38 |
| Network TV | 13 |
| Cable TV | 10 |
| Internet | 5 |

Reprinted with permission of Aspen Publishers, Inc. from R. Coile, *Health Trends*. July 1999; 11(9):5, Table 2. Data originally presented at a conference: Hisle M. Information marketplace megatrends. Superior Consultant, presentation materials, Reno, NV, May 7, 1999.

capture this large potential group of patients. Table 10–1 shows how many years it took different primary communications media to become accepted by 50 million users in this country. This figure highlights how quickly the Internet has been assimilated into the mainstream compared to other commonly used channels.

The present status of health care provider websites does not exceed the introductory level, and many sites experience fewer than expected hits, short visits, and an infrequent number of return visits. The overwhelming reason for this situation often is that sites are haphazardly assembled, too busy, and lack value or useful information for patients. A recent poll of Internet shoppers by e-BuyersGuide.com revealed that 13% of those people would not return to a site because they were dissatisfied with what the site offered.[5] Do you really need a website? The Arthur Anderson company estimated that, at the beginning of the millennium, no less than 36% of all the small businesses in the United States would have a website and that 10–30% of their revenue would be generated by the Internet.[6] Additional support shows that, in 1996, the number of small businesses on-line in the United States was 8% but, by the end of year 2000, it was expected to quintuple to 41%.[7]

A Consumer Technology Survey, performed by PricewaterhouseCoopers at the end of 1998, found the Internet had an estimated $1.7 billion in sales that year; and respondents stated they were comfortable spending an average of $295 per purchase, a figure well within the target price range of the ECP setting.[8]

The demographics of the Internet closely mirror the residential and small to mid-sized business categories. Individual Internet shoppers have mean incomes of $50,000 to $75,000 and use the Internet to re-search goods and services. Web users are also extremely prone to turn-over. By their nature, on-line customers are savvy comparison shoppers who will readily jump to the provider offering the better price, newest feature or other inducement.[7]

Hyperlinks, meta tags, key words, search engines, spiders, banners, on-line chats, and events are just part of the vocabulary specific to this relatively new, enormous, and limitless marketing media.[9] When developing your website, a few general sugges-tions are to avoid sound, movement, blinks, and color change; use only one GIF (graphic interchange format) per page; avoid large graphic images; register your site with major search engines; refine "meta tags" and "swap links"; and place your website address (uniform resource locator) on your business cards, spectacle cases, and all print media you use.[10] Include "what's in it for me" information, not just an office sales pitch.

## E-Commerce

The International Trade Administration has defined *e-commerce* as "any activity that utilizes some form of electronic communication in the inventory, exchange, advertisement, distribution and pay-ment for goods and services."[11] This includes transactions of a commercial nature that use Internet websites or e-mail to transfer information or offer products and services either to other busi-nesses or directly to consumers. This accounts for all forms of com-mercial transactions based on the transmission of digitized data, including text, sound, and visual images. Do you ask for patients' e-mail addresses on your initial patient history forms? Do you have a space where they can affirm if they wish to receive elec-tronic updates your office will send out on the latest developments in vision and ocular health-related issues?

E-commerce has three goals: to improve practice financial performance, to improve service delivery, and to enhance patient education.[12] The maximum e-commerce capability that the Internet offers will not be realized until access is nearly universal, computer skills are much better understood by users, systems become more compatible, and patients are more willing to share financial data on-line.[13] This delay in Internet literacy by potential patients offers the ECP a window of opportunity to prepare for a possible rush on e-commerce as an accepted business channel. Futurist Adam Toffler, author of *Future Shock* and the *Third Wave*, claims that "if you have a company and you're not moving toward automation on demand, you'll have a competitor one day soon who will put you out of business."[14]

Internet technology allows patients to locate the best prices by researching products, comparing prices, and checking availability, empowering patients to expect better service from providers. Websites such as bottomdollar.com or comparenet.com allow patients to compare the prices and features of virtually any product including contact lenses and spectacle frames. Forrester Research estimates that 9 million families spent $8 billion on on-line purchases in 1998, and by 2003, more than 50 million families are expected to spend an excess of $100 billion.[15] Patients will have increasing leverage in the future. The ECP as retailer must understand how to adjust to higher levels of consumer knowledge and buying power. "Shop 'til you drop' has gone to 'drop shopping.' Consumers have little patience for retailers that do not understand them or refuse to adapt their business practices to today's lifestyles."[8]

## Reasons to Have a Website

Net relations is a new marketing communications discipline that combines traditional direct marketing and public relations using the Internet.[3] The idea is to deliver information directly to the target audience or attract them to a particular website by creating added value, either through additional benefit or lower cost. The goal is to increase the confidence patients have in their expectations that they will gain unique or superior value by buying from you and using your services. You also can instill a higher level of confidence that patients indeed receive the highest possible value, eliminating any doubts patients have and confirming your services are superior in value to competitors.[16]

Practice websites should "provide value through their on-line services in addition to interactive functions such as product introductions and customer service. Targeted and value added products are seen as necessities in order to fully realize the potential of marketing strategies through the Internet."[17] According to Michael Tchong, editor of *Iconocast*, an e-mail newsletter, web marketing offers "predictive service" capability, the next phase in business.[18] The Internet makes keeping track of customers easier by allowing ECPs to add a personal touch to their websites, show products to patients that they are interested in buying, and gather information from surveys that rank patient likes and dislikes based on the answers to a few questions.[10] Table 10–2 indicates a few of the many ways ECPs can use the Internet to their advantage.[19]

When the wholesale price of a product is known by patients and is readily available from several sources, it becomes a commodity. By default, the most successful strategy that applies to the sale of commodity products is lowest-cost provider. One way to strengthen the ECPs position is to enhance the patient's knowledge and understanding about products by using new retail sales strategy that offer patient convenience. Marketing and communicating with patients through the Internet enhances the doctor-patient relationship.

A study found the biggest challenges in maintaining a website were keeping up with the technology (21%), keeping the site

**Table 10–2   Internet Uses**

1. Welcome patients, explain policies (have receptionist refer to site).
2. Answer vision and eye health questions.
3. Educate and inform patients, employers, referral sources.
4. Expanded brochure capable of listing services offered, a history of the practice and information about the ECPs and staff personnel.
5. Provide directions for traveling to the facility with maps and photos.
6. Enable professional consults.
7. Conduct on-line market research, patient surveys, and opinion polls.
8. Recall and appointment reminders.
9. Schedule appointments and order products.

current (21%), finding time to work on it (14%), obtaining internal support (5%), and recruiting talent to work on the site (5%).[19] Objectives in using the Internet for marketing ranged from communication (17%), followed by providing information (16%), obtaining referrals (16%), building awareness (16%), educating patients and providers (5%), and building an Internet presence (5%).[19] One area needing attention concerned the methods for evaluating the effectiveness and return on investment. Less than 20% evaluated their Internet investment. The majority simply used number of visitors (67%), followed by referrals generated from the site (27%), and patient surveys (7%). When asked "How important do you expect the Internet to become in marketing health care within the next five years?," nearly 80% responded it will become important.[19]

Another compelling reason to develop Internet capabilities is the growing number of third-party payers and government agencies requiring businesses to submit claims for reimbursement using electronic data interchange (EDI). In the near future, it is quite possible that managed care organizations (MCOs) and health plans will connect patient inquiries to provider offices through hyperlinks. As an ECP, you would not want to miss the opportunity of gaining access to potential patients who are seeking eyecare through Internet searches of their health plan's database. The following questions will help you decide if it is right for you to have an Internet presence:[20]

1. Can I offer additional services or information to existing patients?
2. Can I serve new groups of patients by modifying my current information?
3. Can I develop new sources of revenue?
4. Will I lose revenue to my competitors if I have no Internet presence?

Three reasons why health care providers do not use the Internet are lack of desire or sophistication in the use of technology, dislike for new methods of communication (technophobia), and unwillingness to change their personal attitude about sharing information, knowledge, and experience in a new way.[21] However, professional on-line user groups offer advantages to ECPs that include sharing professional experiences, distributing firsthand information, and the opportunity to discuss common problems. These are primary reasons why market research reveals regular Internet usage by physicians has tripled in the past two years.[22]

## Development Stages of an Eyecare Website

The developmental stages of eyecare websites can be classified into the following distinct categories:[23]

> Level 1. Electronic text, sound, graphics, and motion.
> Level 2. Addition of map link, vendor links, site entertainment, and e-mail.
> Level 3. Basic interactivity, product ordering and appointment scheduling, patient opinion polls and surveys, updated insurance information.
> Level 4. E-commerce transaction capability and user customization, site search engines and drop-down menus.

### Level 1

Level 1 consists only of text, sound, graphics, and motion. The site content might include a statement about the philosophy of the practice, public service information about consumer vision, a description of office personnel, hours of operation, billing policies, directions, vision plans accepted, and products and services offered. The website pages are permanent, fixed presentations taking a broad communication approach with no interactivity or incentives offered to revisit the site. An example of a Level 1 index web page is shown in Figure 10–1.

### Level 2

Level 2 web pages are expanded, with content that might include cyber-tours of the office; comprehensive and detailed explanations

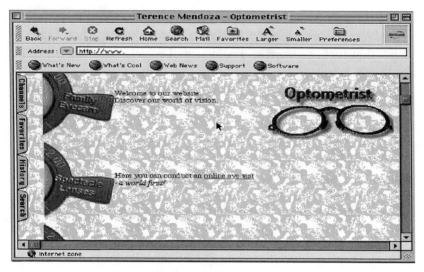

**Figure 10–1   Level 1 index page.**

of services offered; biographies or curriculum vitaes of the practice providers. Additionally, the site may include cross-referenced information that is either cumbersome or rapidly changing and impractical to print. This website can offer current information that can be rapidly and inexpensively modified, unlike printed material. Hyperlinks can be offered to outside patient education or health-related sites of interest, as well as links to map sites and vendors offering consumer information. E-mail can be added as a basic channel of communication. An example of a Level 2 web page showing travel directions to the practice using a map link is shown in Figure 10–2.

### Level 3

The Level 3 site offers the start of basic real-time interactive capabilities, including scheduling an appointment and ordering products. The site content offers the patient advanced capabilities such as surveys and specialized forms providing the practice with patient feedback and requests for information. Market research and patient surveys performed using Internet websites offer ECPs the ability to obtain the most accurate, current patient feedback about their services. This speed and quality of informa-

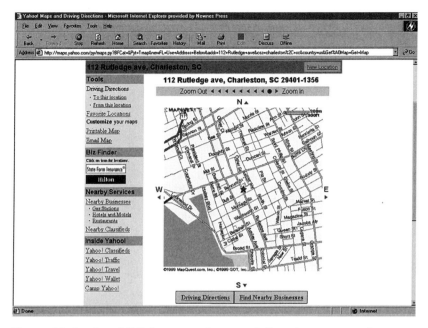

**Figure 10–2   Level 2 link to map for travel directions to practice.**

tion offer an immeasurable advantage in making important business decisions. The two components of traditional market research with the highest cost are data collection and analysis.[24] Using a web-based survey eliminates the need for interviewers, greatly reducing the cost of data collection. Site characteristics include active patient involvement, which creates a reason to return, and customized surveys to allow the provider to collect marketing data about patients and inform patients about special offers. Figures 10–3 and 10–4 show interactive services that are made convenient for the patient through the use of web pages.

## Level 4

Drop-down menus and search engines permit the user to maneuver and customize the search on demand. Web page content allows patients to update personal information and offers on-line chat capability and e-commerce transaction capability that requires site security and encryption coding for patient protection. These highly sophisticated sites include the ability to create cus-

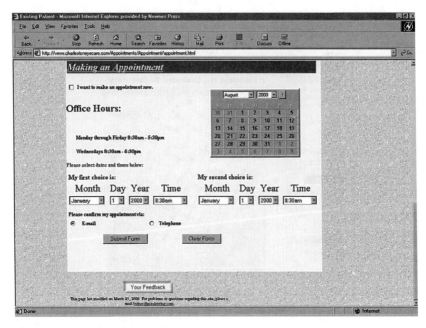

**Figure 10–3    Level 3 making an appointment.**

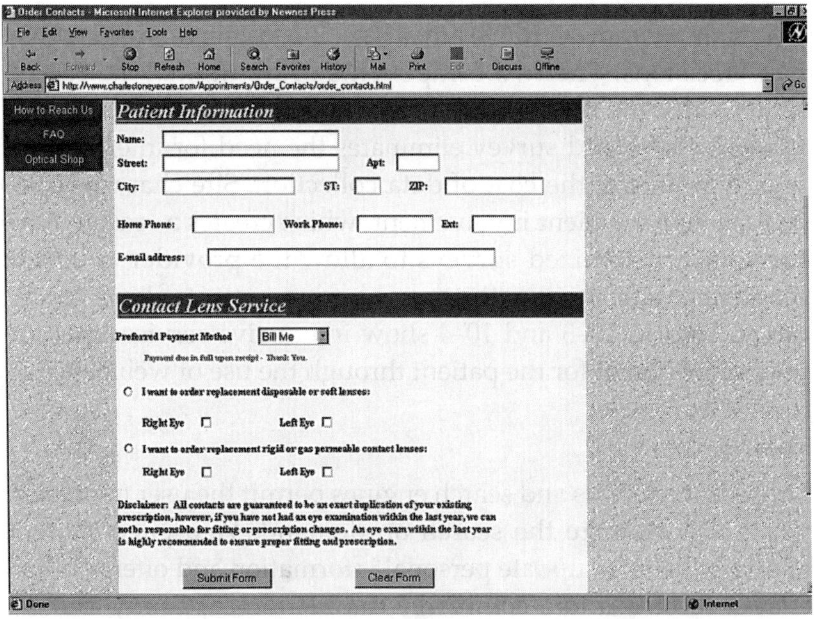

**Figure 10–4    Level 3 ordering a product.**

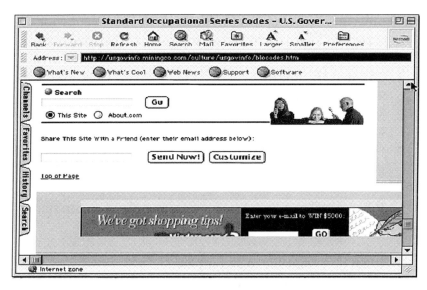

**Figure 10–5    Level 4 site visitor customization.**

tomized patient databases, allowing the office to collect individualized specific information used for segmenting and targeting markets and the ability to recognize return visitors while retaining previous interactive information. The ability to offer e-commerce to patients is facilitated by the use of e-cash, a concept being tested in select markets, using software such as Mondex, CyberCash, and CyberCoin.[25] Major innovators of this new technology are CyberCash, Inc., in Reston, Virginia, and DigiCash in San Mateo, California. Figure 10–5 shows a web page that offers patients the ability to customize to their needs.

Levels 1 and 2 site visitors are potential customers looking for information; your function should be to inform them by emphasizing awareness of your services. You can enhance the doctor-patient relationship by providing easy access to practice information. Levels 3 and 4 require serious financial and personnel commitment and planning on how the site fits into your practice objectives. Improved patient relations can be achieved if sites are created that address specific patient needs, resulting in increased repeat patient visits. Methods of gaining patient response include opinion polls, bulletin boards, surveys, and on-line patient focus group chats.[26]

Consumer Internet health care resources are one avenue for the ECP to explore for expanded Internet presence. These include

1. "Annual Healthcare Guide to the Internet," COR Resources Santa Barbara, California.
2. Medical World Search (www.mwsearch.com), the largest health care search site.
3. Health on the Net Foundation (www.hon.ch) certifies sites that meet consumer health care information standards.

When developing your web marketing plan you can start by answering these questions:

1. What do I want site to accomplish?
2. Who do I want to visit the site?
3. What are my target markets?
4. What type of practice information would these targets value?
5. What do I want site visitors to be able to do?

## Getting Started Using the Web

The first step in the creation of a practice website is to decide on the specific objectives you want your site to accomplish. Do you want to make more potential patients aware of what your practice offers? Do you want to use your site to add to the uniqueness of your practice relative to your competitors? The next step is to assign specific personnel responsibility for specific aspects of website development. You must allocate adequate resources for the selected staff member to obtain any required skills he or she cannot perform. This responsibility can be outsourced if no internal personnel can achieve the desired results. However, this option can be costlier and possibly riskier due to less direct control.

After a staff member has been identified, determine the target patient groups and set priorities on the type of information you want each different group to receive. In this way, you can separate high-priority information for general as well as specialty patient groups. Also, the hyperlinks to be established with outside resources should be identified. Test the different types of information and links to see how well each meets the objectives you want to achieve and eliminate or change those deemed less likely to accomplish desired results. Send out notices to patients that your website is up and running, post notices in your office, and have your receptionist tell patients at sign-in about the site. "The key to a successful Website is making it dynamic. Information needs to be changed and added on a regular basis. Otherwise repeat traffic will not occur."[27] Finally, the methods to measure the effectiveness of your efforts, which can be quite difficult, should be chosen; the number of hits per month and number of patient inquiries generated from the site are two commonly used methods.

A well-designed, web-based selling strategy addresses the future by collecting information about patients and website visitors. Web-visitor "click prints" are collected for market trends, based on patient inquiries and searches of your site. An analysis of these "click prints," including point of origin, length of time spent, and services searched, offers a detailed picture of the interests of site visitors.[28] Using new web forecasting technology will allow you to develop and deliver a variety of messages and web content directly to inquiring potential patients. ECPs should become familiar with customer segmentation, profiling, and predictive modeling. With this knowledge, you can develop and implement targeted programs.

Many of the marketing tasks delegated to office personnel can be successfully performed by the use of a database and your website. Human effort can be replaced by the "hard technology" of equipment or by improving work processes through the "soft technology" of applications.[29] Should you decide to outsource the development of your marketing web pages, in addition to accepting a predetermined price to develop your web pages, this form of media has several new and innovative approaches that can be used to price the creation of your website, including cost per visitor, cost per transaction, or cost per patient acquisition.[30]

To the Internet user and surfer "free attracts." Giveaways keep website visitors lured.[25] Entertainment is a great attraction and interest holder of web users. Have them enter their e-mail address to win a discount on a featured eyewear product or a gift certificate for future use. Regularly scheduled contests may entice visitors to return to your site often. According to a May 1999 survey conducted by New York City research firm Jupiter Communications, 76% of web surfers surveyed liked sweepstakes-style prize giveaways, many of which were announced using banner advertising from other websites.[31] One word of caution: Should you choose to use giveaways or sweepstakes, make sure you include a visible, concise privacy statement. The Federal Trade Commission is cracking down on Internet scams, and awareness of the laws governing this form of enticement is essential.

Other options are to offer free computer-generated acuity screenings or list warning signs of visual problems as well as links to interesting educational and complimentary pages. And don't forget to post testimonials from satisfied, enthusiastic patients. Ask for a credit card only if your site is protected with encryption technology, otherwise offer a toll-free phone number. View your site using different browsers and monitor size to make sure the visual balance is the same for different formats. Finally, once your website is operational, make sure to inform as many search engines and directories as possible. This way when potential patients are searching indexes, your practice will be a prominent link that is easily contacted, as shown in Figure 10–6. Web marketing resources to visit for ideas include

www.iconbazaar.com (shareware).
www.websitesthatsuck.com (web page ideas).
www.webcrawler.com, then search "marketing tools."
www.quackwatch.com (health care fraud and decision making).

## Present Status of Eyecare Websites— A Research Survey

A research survey limited to eyecare office websites was performed in February and March 2000 by six third-year students at

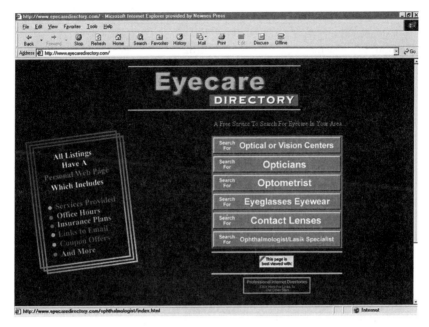

**Figure 10–6    Search engine directory.**

the New England College of Optometry and overseen by one of the authors.[32] The keywords searched were limited to optometrists, ophthalmologists, and opticians. Only websites of practices were included in the survey. We did not include sites that had laser vision as the keyword or primary offering, although these particular sites typically are more advanced, Level 2 or 3, and better developed. The search also was limited by time constraints to Yahoo, Northern Lights, Alta Vista, and AOL. We found 60% of optometric practices and 95% of ophthalmology practices that have websites contain at least five web pages, while only 35% of optician offices have more than five web pages. Table 10–3 offers details of the survey from which the following conclusions can be drawn as of mid-2000: First, it is evident from the results that the vast majority of websites are in the introductory phase, offering tremendous opportunity for short-term future development. Second, there is great opportunity for practices to form alliances and find corporate sponsors via links and banners as a source of consumer information, site embellishment, and possibly revenue. Third, in many

## Table 10–3   Sample Size

|  | ODs (%) | OMDs (%) | Opticians (%) |
|---|---|---|---|
| *Site Sections* | | | |
| About this practice | 82 | 62 | 36 |
| Description of personnel | 57 | 83 | 0 |
| Tour of office | 6 | 3 | 0 |
| Frequently asked questions | 46 | 34 | 5 |
| Information about spectacles | 51 | 16 | 55 |
| Information about contact lenses | 54 | 16 | 16 |
| Information about laser vision | 34 | 63 | 0 |
| Information about ocular health | 52 | 47 | 3 |
| Directions to office | 10 | 52 | 3 |
| Map or map link | 54 | 5 | 41 |
| Update patient insurance information | 5 | 0 | 3 |
| *Interactivity* | | | |
| E-mail | 74 | 75 | 61 |
| Make an appointment | 8 | 2 | 0 |
| Order product | 3 | 0 | 9 |
| Pay for product | 0 | 1 | 7 |
| Search engine | 0 | 4 | 1 |
| Drop-down menu | 1 | 0 | 0 |
| Search personal information | 1 | 0 | 0 |
| *Present Level of Site* | | | |
| 1 | 48 | 92 | 70 |
| 2 | 46 | 5 | 23 |
| 3 | 6 | 3 | 5 |
| 4 | 0 | 0 | 0 |
| *Offsite Links to* | | | |
| Frame manufacturers | 3 | 3 | 20 |
| Spectacle lens manufacturers | 6 | 3 | 7 |
| Contact lens manufacturers | 3 | 3 | 7 |
| Professional vision organizations | 22 | 24 | 5 |
| Consumer education organizations | 35 | 14 | 18 |
| *Outside Links* | | | |
| None | 48 | 71 | 77 |
| 1 | 8 | 3 | 5 |
| 2–5 | 27 | 10 | 9 |
| 6–14 | 16 | 10 | 2 |
| Over 15 | 1 | 6 | 7 |
| *Webpages* | | | |
| 1 | 34 | 3 | 20 |
| 2–4 | 6 | 0 | 45 |
| 5–8 | 27 | 55 | 33 |
| 9–14 | 29 | 42 | 2 |
| Over 15 | 2 | 0 | 0 |

ODs: $n = 93$     OMDs: $n = 129$     Opticians: $n = 44$
All numbers are in percentages.

cases, it was difficult and time consuming to find practice websites. There is a need to differentiate practice sites and better index sites to facilitate patient access. The ability for a site to offer keyword searches at this point in time is available but probably is not cost effective. However, within the next three years, as more specialized web hosting develops, more sophisticated services will become available, making it easier, less expensive, and time saving for the ECP to have a practice website.

## Database Marketing

Database marketing is a system that combines information about patients and their purchase history with software offering insight into strategic marketing questions of importance, such as which products sell best, which brands are most profitable, and what time of year is best to concentrate on selling specific products. The goal of database marketing is to increase the effectiveness and efficiency of your practice's communication by targeting existing patients, developing leads to attract new patients, and influencing patient behavior whether it be with compliance issues, return visits, or purchases. One advantage is that it allows you to develop a close, informed, flexible relationship with your patients no matter what your goals are, whether to augment your patient base, increase sales of a new product or service, or expand repeat business. Desired results can best be achieved by "amassing large quantities of customer data in computerized form and then massaging the information to pinpoint the best customers and target them in a more personal way."[33] Most eyecare businesses have some type of electronic patient filing system, but simply having lists of names in a computer does not mean you have a true marketing database.[34] One physician uses database mailing to send annual health status reports to his patients. He took the idea from his accountant from whom he received a report on the progress of his financial worth during the past year.[35]

Conventional external mass marketing, on the other hand, places emphasis on new patient acquisition. Research cited in the chapter on developing an eyecare marketing identity indicates costs of five times or greater to acquire a new patient as compared to retaining existing patients. This is where database marketing has a distinct advantage, by improving revenue through analysis of present patient spending patterns and needs. The value of using database marketing is in patient retention and maximizing the benefits received from establishing long-term patient relationships.

The advantage of database marketing rests in the ability to target patients whose known interests and past buying behavior predicts a higher probability of acceptance or use of your services. Another value-added use can be found during the period after a new patient makes an appointment and prior to the actual visit. "Whenever there is information the significance of which the provider of the service knows far better than the customer, there is an opportunity to proactively promote satisfaction, i.e. reduce negative and enhance positive aspects of their first experience."[36]

The primary function of database marketing is to increase revenue by customizing service to frequent consumers, formulating offerings to specific segments, and augmenting buyer purchasing behavior. A secondary goal is to continually upgrade and enhance your database as a future revenue resource. Traditional mass market image ads (newspaper, radio, mailers) can enhance your practice name or brand awareness but do not necessarily result in sales. Direct database marketing is designed to elicit a response through leads, inquiries, or sales. Another advantage of database marketing is the ability to track costs, the number of responses, and revenue generated, making it easier for you to determine the cost-effectiveness of various media tactics used.

Specific types of database marketing include[36]

1. Frequency marketing is used to increase the number of times a patient buys a specific product by suggesting additional uses; for example, one-day contact lenses for sports or social events.
2. Cross marketing is used to increase the range of products a patient buys; for example, computer comfort Rx spectacles.

3. Upmarketing upgrades patients to more expensive premium products; for example, by applying benefits allowed to the total cost and emphasizing the savings over the full cost.

## Using Databases in Eyecare Practices

Until very recently, health care databases have been restricted in their ability to utilize data and customize patient messages, limited to traditional data such as name, age, address, phone, and previous purchase history. The use of segmentation allows the ECP's office to identify and target specific patient groups based on similar characteristics within any one particular group or dissimilarities among various groups. Using print media, variable printing takes this process one step further, allowing the insertion of text, names, and addresses "into designated fields within a generic piece of marketing."[37]

The first step to take when deciding to utilize database marketing is to determine what you want to achieve, the information and resources required, and how you must change your staff's attitude to successfully incorporate this new system of patient communication. Successful database marketing is not a technology issue. The emphasis is on your operational efficiency, systems and processes in place, and your attitude, not the technology, which simply is a tool that enables you to market and predict trends easier and faster.[38] Make sure you understand how you will use the data you collect. What information do you need that is not readily available? How can you obtain it and at what intervals do you need to update it? Develop a system for staff members talking with patients to take notes on the conversation. This will help you learn which "hot buttons" are on patient's minds, then at a later time, enter those comments in the computer.[39] In the future, you or your staff can do a search for any key words or phrases made by patients.

Determine the most effective ways to stay in contact with patients. Patient loyalty offers the most reliable method of predicting future profits. It is essential that the right message using the medium with the highest probability of reaching the right patient is delivered at the right time. Direct marketing is not direct mail or telemarketing. Direct marketing integrates several different media, taking into account all costs incurred. A major advantage of database marketing is its ability to track costs. A marketing database is part of an integrated marketing model that justifies all costs.[38]

Commonly used examples of database marketing include biannual reminders to contact lens patients, follow-up letters to refractive surgery patients, referral letters to personnel benefits administrators, and birthday cards to current patients. Annual exam recall can be developed using a database and age as a segmenting factor. Create reminders using messages and themes that are relevant to various age groups. This strengthens your relationship with patients because each age group will perceive that your practice image appeals to it. The quality of your data can be constantly assessed and updated, simply by tracking the percentage of returned mail from every mailing. If more than 4% of your mail is returned for bad addresses, it is an indication that your mailing list is not as current as it should be and needs to be updated.[34]

When buying database management software ask what database capabilities are included, how simple is it to use, and how adaptable is it for future changes. When shopping for software remember you should understand its content, not format, before you begin to look for a program. A few questions to answer when shopping for software are these:[39]

1. How many customizable fields will I require for each patient?
2. How easy will it be for staff to input information?
3. What format will allow the easiest interpretation of the information reports?
4. Can the finished reports be customized for my needs?

## Sources of Practice Information

The information used to develop your patient databases comes from several sources. Patient responses to in-person office, telephone, or mail surveys can be combined with the information found in patient files, written history questionnaires, and from e-mail or website postings to create "patient profiles."[33] These profiles then can be merged with your chosen marketing mix to send personalized messages to patients about treatment regimens, side effects, recalls, and reminder appointments as well as motivational material and warnings about lifestyle issues related to noncompliance. The customized messages can be delivered by direct mail, phone, or the Internet through e-mail. Since previous behavior usually is the best and most reliable predictor of future behavior, when targeting previous patients, the most useful information to use is RFM: recentness of purchase, frequency of purchase, and monetary amount of purchase.[40]

Databases containing information specific to an individual patient's needs, interests, or lifestyle requirements allows the ECP to standardize the various components involved in communicating with these patients and marketing products or services to satisfy their individual needs. Once the database is initiated, the ECP can establish guidelines, standards, and measuring criteria for the types of messages the office sends, their frequency, and patient responses received. A database of standard responses to frequently asked questions allows the ECP's employees to respond faster and uniformly to patient questions, reducing the possibility of inappropriate or different information given to different patients asking the same question. This eliminates wasted time, frees up ECP's time, and limits the number of questions a staff member must respond to without the guidance of a preprogrammed "expert" database as assistance.[41]

Define and acquire only information that you feel is essential. When deciding what data to add to your database, be extremely selective or you will collect too much valueless information. Limit your input of data to what you believe is required to perform and measure marketing programs within the next two years.

## Assessing Database Marketing Effectiveness

To assess how effective your database marketing program is, monitor three parameters to measure the return on your efforts and changes in patients' attitudes, behavior, and spending patterns.[42]

First, feedback from patients about changes in attitude should inform you about the extent of the impact on patients' opinions. Measurements should include patient awareness of your marketing program and individual patient likes or dislikes. In addition, tabulate the changes in patient acceptance or rejection of various brand products and how this effects your business image. Second, behavioral changes in patient spending patterns can be detected by collecting data that specifies the number of patient inquiries for a new product or service, the change in percentage of volume for new product offerings, and the amount of incremental business that has been generated by the marketing program. Third, determine the marketing program's financial performance compared to other programs. Develop patient profiles and seek reasons why a marketing outcome occurred. For example, why did a particular mailing coupon or announcement work? Did it result in a large number of new inquiries or patients substituting one brand for another? Once you have analyzed results from these three areas of your database program, you will know what changes or new directions to take. The quality of your database can be evaluated using different parameters, which include[43]

1. *Addressability.* How easy is it to identify and reach each patient segment?
2. *Measurability.* Can your data reveal the frequency of usage of services by each segment, including when and why individuals use your services?
3. *Flexibility.* Can your data appeal in different ways and at different times?
4. *Accountability.* Does your database contain data that will be profitable?

## Things to Avoid While Using the Net

Problems have surfaced in the area of customer service related to Internet marketing that you will want to avoid. A recent report revealed that 23% of on-line users who experienced problems in 1999 shopping on the Internet, no longer use the Internet to make purchases.[44] Another area of concern is inadequate service, in the form of not replying to inquiries in a timely manner. A study by Jupiter Communications showed that only 59% of 125 of the most prominent sites in the areas of content, travel, retail, financial services, and consumer brands responded to e-mail within two days.[45] Several businesses have lost the opportunities offered by the web to enhance personal relationships with consumers by not following through with customer service.

There is a growing resistance by consumers to provide information for commercial purposes. The market research industry is concerned with dropping rates of consumer responses when asked to participate in quantitative surveys. A study reported in *Shopping Futures* found that only 50% of consumers are willing to provide personal information to businesses, down from over 60% in 1995.[46] Consumers were willing to release information only to businesses they trusted and with which they were familiar. The majority of respondents were happy to provide personal details if the result was a better product or service.[46] In the near future, it may become necessary for businesses doing patient-centered market research to offer incentives encouraging people to provide data.

The third area to avoid is exaggerated claims and false advertising. The federal government has yet to develop new regulations on Internet advertising, however, the Federal Trade Commission (FTC) has started to monitor Internet advertising content. Several instances of misleading and false claims have been investigated. One high-profile case involved claims about contact lenses.[47] This involved assertions about the results of orthokeratology as a substitute for refractive surgery. The site owners eventually made changes conforming to FTC recommendations. To comply with accepted practices of health-related advertising, The Health On the Net Foundation has developed a set of principles to assist those interested in health-related marketing on the Internet. Also, the American Medical Association has released guidelines to help ensure the reliability and accuracy of website content while protecting patient confidentiality.[48]

A predetermined database marketing campaign does have a few shortcomings.[49] First, it doesn't always take into account the patient purchasing cycle. Database marketing campaigns often start with a fixed calendar of marketing tactics and strategies based on prior years' results, with additions made based on the introduction of new products and services. Next, the ECP chooses specific products and services to include in any promotion patients are targeted to receive. Rather than choosing targeted patients after the ECP has created the marketing campaign, it makes more sense and offers a better return on investment to develop campaigns to fit patients' needs. Predetermined patient targets eliminate potentially valuable segments that may not receive sufficient marketing communications.

## Recent Advances

Software has recently been developed that can "profile" visitors to your website using "collaborative filtering," a technique that gives your site the capability to offer selective viewing to your patients and present customized images and text pertinent to each individual.[50] Profiling will allow the ECP's website to personalize and revise viewer content immediately on a real-time basis. Additionally, patterns of patient purchase or inquiry can be determined through a technique called *data mining.*[51] These patterns of patient behavior often are undetectable without the use of the sophisticated software that places every distinct piece of information in its own table to avoid repetition, a technique known as *indexing.*[37] For example, data may be tabulated on a last name basis and sorted by phone number. In this case, both last name and phone number become index terms. Any deviations based on expected or previous experience can be used to anticipate future trends in patient behavior and needs.[38]

Another advance in database marketing is found with interactive communication technology, allowing the user to distinguish differences among patients and produce messages for individual patients. In general, database marketing methods become costlier and less practical to utilize as the ECP's message to individual patients becomes more personalized.[33] Traditional database marketing can identify differences among individuals but it cannot create separate pieces for each of them. "Interactive communication technology tailors content—layout, design, words, sentences, paragraphs and graphics—ensuring that each piece is totally unique, created for a particular individual and no one else."[33] Another development that enhances the relationship practices have with patients is found in customer relationship management (CRM) technology. This new application allows the user to integrate all patient data into one system that is totally customer centered. The four main principles of CRM are:[52]

1. Identify your patients.
2. Differentiate their needs and their value to your practice.
3. Interact with them in cost-efficient ways that enhance your service effectiveness.
4. Customize portions of the products or services you offer patients.

The interaction that results from CRM should produce "information that can help you strengthen and deepen your customer relationships"[53] by the ECP learning how to better satisfy patients.

It is estimated that, by the year 2002, the demand for this technology will increase tenfold and may set the standard by which businesses communicate with customers.[54] Today's marketing buzzwords that emanate from customer relationship management include focus, one-to-one targeting, and mass customization. In addition to incorporating marketing science, the ECP's programs require creativity and imaginative thinking. Danish philosopher, Rolf Jensen forecasts "the Dream Society will soon replace the Information Age, ushering in a market definition that is more grounded on emotions."[55]

## Action Plan for ECPs

1. Recognize how the Internet can enhance your marketing capabilities.
2. Register your practice domain name.
3. Collect patient e-mail addresses and consider revising your practice patient questionnaire to gather this data.

4. Survey other eyecare websites to determine your preferences.
5. Compile sources of website developers to investigate when you are ready to start your own practice website.

## Notes

1. Brown E. 9 ways to win on the Web. *Fortune.* May 24, 1999: 112.
2. News broadcast segment on WBZ 1030 AM, Boston, at 3:25 P.M. on September 3, 1999.
3. Spataro M. Net relations: A fusion of direct marketing and public relations. *Direct Marketing.* August 1998;61(4):16–19.
4. Gallaga O. Internet gives cancer patients information. *Knight-Ridder Tribune Business News,* on-line article, February 8, 1999:1–3.
5. Rosenberg R. Shoppers in poll report service dissatisfaction. *Boston Globe.* September 8, 1999:D4.
6. Wrestling with the web. *Business Week.* May 24, 1999:16.
7. Rubin C. Mom 'n' pop stores learn how worldwide the web really is. *USA Weekend.* December 17–19, 1999:4.
8. The medium is the message. *Telephony.* November 23, 1998: ISSN 0040-2656.
9. Furchott R. It's a honey of a website, but where's the buzz. *Business Week.* October 12, 1998:ENT4.
10. Design a better website. *Journal of Accountancy.* August 1998; 186(2):181.
11. Campbell A. Ten reasons why your business should use electronic commerce. *Business America.* May 1998;119(5):12–15.
12. Gerber P, Bijlefeld M. Aim is reducing costs of doing business. *EyeWorld.* March 2000:62.
13. Coile R. Health care e-commerce and the Internet. *Health Trends.* July 1999;11(9):5.
14. Toffler: Change—or else. *Inc.* May 1998;20(6):23.
15. Loewe P, Bonchek M. The retail revolution. *Management Review.* April 1999:38.
16. MacStravic S. Marketing by means of the confidence factor. *Health Care Strategic Management.* January 1998:19–23.

17. Hoey C. Maximizing the effectiveness of web-based marketing communications. *Marketing Intelligence and Planning.* January–February 1998;16(1):31.
18. Feuerstein A. E-commerce gets personal. *San Francisco Business Times.* April 16, 1999;13(37):1–2.
19. Shepherd D, Fell D. Marketing on the Internet. *Journal of Health Care Marketing.* Winter 1995;15(4):12–16.
20. Ghosh S. Making business sense of the Internet. *Harvard Business Review.* March–April 1998:126–135.
21. Shepherd D, Fell D. Hospital marketing and the Internet. *Journal of Health Care Marketing.* Winter 1996;16(4):47–48.
22. Healtheon. Physician use of the Internet explodes. *Health Management Technology.* March 20, 1999;20(2):8.
23. Suggested from a discussion in Shepherd C, Fell D. Building websites that attract visitors. *Marketing Health Services.* Spring 1998:44–45.
24. McCollugh D. Web-based market research: The dawning of a new age. *Direct Marketing.* December 1998;61(18):36–38.
25. Gregg L. Will you be ready for e-cash? *Credit Union Executive.* January–February 1998;38(1):12–14.
26. Kirsner S. Listen up. *CIO.* April 1, 1998;11(12):24–25.
27. Widmer T, Shepherd C. Developing a hospital website as a marketing tool. *Marketing Health Services.* Spring 1999:32–33.
28. Stevens T. Set sale on the "Net." *Industry Week.* April 21, 1997;246(8):56–67.
29. Leavitt T. Industrialization of service. *Harvard Business Review.* September–October 1976:63–74.
30. McHale T. Having your tea and drinking it too. *Brandweek.* May 24, 1999;40(21):28.
31. Fryer B. Let's make a deal: Website promotions are the bait to hook sales. *Your Company.* October 1, 1999;9(7):94.
32. Our research assistants were Neha Ashar, Ann Bennett, Stacy Friedman, Dimple Nanchahal, Ilaxi Rani, and Robert Sholomon.
33. Field A. Precision marketing. *Inc.* June 18, 1996;18(9):54–58.
34. Carey M. Marketing databases: So near and yet so far. *Direct Marketing.* November 1998;61(7):26–29.

35. Baker S. *Managing Patient Expectations*. San Francisco: Jossey-Bass; 1998:251.
36. MacStravic S. We're missing the boat in database marketing. *Marketing Health Services*. Summer 1998:39–42.
37. Reeves C, Bulger D. Database marketing: Reaching an audience of one. *Behavioral Health Management*. January 1999; 19(1):42.
38. Poulos N. Twelve database marketing principles—Part 1. *Target Marketing*. September 1997;20(9):46–49.
39. Poulos N. Implementing a plan—Part 2. *Target Marketing*. October 1997;20(10):100–102.
40. Ables G. Predictive modeling for non-statisticians. *Target Marketing*. March 1997;20(3):14–15.
41. Bohl D, ed. *Close to the Customer, An American Management Research Report on Consumer Affairs*. New York: American Management Association; 1987:49.
42. Hess M, Mayer B. Test and evaluate your way to success. *Marketing News*. July 5, 1999;33(14):12.
43. Vavra T. The database marketing imperative. *Direct Marketing*. Winter 1993;2(1):46.
44. DeLong S. Net not a bed of roses. *Eyecare Business*. May 2000: 16.
45. Lidsky D. The service you deserve. *PC Magazine*. October 5, 1999:98.
46. Gofton D. Data firms react to survey fatigue. *Marketing*. April 29, 1999:29–30.
47. Murphy K. Government keeps wary eye on medical advertising on the Net. *Internet World*. October 12, 1998;4(33):15.
48. AMA issues guidelines for medical websites. *The Boston Globe*. March 12, 2000:D15.
49. Bayer J, Heffring P. Less campaign, more customer in calendar plans. *Marketing News*. September 28, 1998;32(20):7.
50. McHugh J. Hall of mirrors. *Forbes*. February 7, 2000:120.
51. Baker K, Baker S. Mine over matter. *Journal of Business Strategy*. July–August 1998;19(4):22–26.
52. A crash course in customer relationship management. *Harvard Management Update*. March 2000;5(3):3–6.

53. Peppers D, Rogers M. *The One-to-One Manager: Lessons in Customer Relationship Management*. New York: Currency/Doubleday; 1999.
54. Miller R. An holistic approach to keeping clients. *Marketing*. July 29, 1999:22–23.
55. Mazur L. Better ditch the figures and use creative instinct. *Marketing*. April 29, 1999:18.

# CHAPTER 11

# Marketing and Valuing the Eyecare Practice for Sale

> *When selling a practice, high gross income is good, but high net income is better.* —G. L. *Moss*

Several key business fundamentals have the greatest effect on the value of an ECP's practice. First, the more prominent the local market position and the more renowned the practice, the easier it is to find a buyer willing to pay a higher price. Second, new regulations affecting reimbursement to providers have an impact on value. Third, more-efficient office operations and systems producing a higher than average net profit margin make it easier to find a buyer willing to pay a higher price. Finally, newer equipment and leasehold improvements that offer more of a turnkey operation add value as well as facilitate the transfer to a new owner.

Factors influencing the local market position are trends in patient volume, ratio of new to former patients, ability to retain former patients, the number and quality of new plans, and associated reimbursement levels. Active ongoing recall, patient communications, and various sources that refer patients to the office also affect value. Managed care changes limiting reimbursement levels and the federal government's Stark II antikickback regulations limiting scope of practice may have a negative impact on final value.

The efficiency of practice operations, including staff ability and eagerness to deliver high-quality service, influences value.

The quality and legibility of patient records and the amount of outstanding collections also influence potential buyers. The cost savings mechanisms employed by the practice and passed on to the patient as part of the value chain and the capability of your information system both affect value.

Assessing your practice in preparation to maximize sale value starts by demonstrating high quality in all phases of patient interaction through a review of office systems. Does the practice deliver cost-effective, high-quality care? Can you document outcomes improvement? Can the practice integrate easily with other practices if needed? Has the seller taken steps to eliminate inappropriate care? Specifically, review patient flow and satisfaction, level of the practice's management information system, type and number of communications and recall messages, ability to schedule an appointment, and the ease that records can be understood by others.

## Practice Appraisal

An appraisal is a useful third party, objective opinion based on education and prior experience; it is a realistic starting point for negotiation. According to Judge David Laro of the U.S. Tax Court, "each valuation case is unique . . . in valuation, there are no absolutes . . . there is no irrefutable right answer . . . experts will and do differ . . . there are available methods that are generally recognized."[1] It is reasonable to expect that an appraisal performed by different appraisers using generally accepted methods should result in values all of which fall within a reasonable range.

The accuracy of any appraisal depends on the appraiser's knowledge, integrity, and experience. The difference between the appraised price and the final sale price varies with the desirability of owning a practice in that particular location, the number of potential buyers, the favorability of financing offered by the seller, the down payment given by the buyer, and the overall history and reputation of the practice. However, the ECP can ask several questions of an appraiser to help evaluate his or her qualifications:[2]

1.  What is your specific education concerning practice or business valuation?

2. How many years and how many appraisals have you performed?
3. Do you do general business appraisal or do you specialize in health care? Specifically, how many eyecare practices have you appraised?
4. Are you certified or licensed in any state?
5. If you perform an appraisal, must you also be hired as a consultant or negotiator.
6. Supply the names of three to five prior clients that you have done work for or represented. I will contact them for possible recommendations or comments.
7. What do you charge and what do I get for that fee? Is this fee for a complete valuation or is there an hourly consultation fee?
8. Have you had any experience or been used previously as an expert witness in court testimony?
9. How many pages are your appraisal reports? How many different methods do you use to value the practice?

## Offering a Proposal

Offering a knowledgeable "sales persona" shows prospective buyers the seller has taken a realistic, determined, proactive stance about the potential transfer of ownership. This can be reinforced by developing a practice sales prospectus, containing specific information detailing the history and finances of the practice, made available to all prospective purchasers and their consultants. This information probably will be requested by all parties seriously interested in the practice and, if assembled, will save a great deal of time during the buyer's phase of prepurchase analysis and decision making, referred to as *due diligence*. The process entails the buyer and his or her consultants and attorney requesting specific legal and financial information to evaluate the practice. Appendix 11–1 lists the relevant information necessary to analyze the value of a practice.[2]

## Due Diligence

Several documents and forms pertaining to the financial and legal aspect of the eyecare business to be transferred should be fully investigated and analyzed by both the purchaser and consultants. The process of uncovering this information is known as *due diligence*. Table 11–1 outlines the material that should be made available. Specific documents include a review of the ownership structure bylaws in the case of professional corporations and shareholder agreements. Is creditor or lender consent required to enter into agreements or transfer assets? Consider obtaining a letter of Assurance or Good Standing with a full disclosure from the seller's attorneys, accountants, and malpractice insurers.

Financial statements that should be reviewed include federal tax returns for the practice, going back 3–5 years; the most

**Table 11–1  Due Diligence**

---

*Corporate/ownership structure.* Review bylaws, shareholder agreements, joint venture relationships, board meeting minutes (if organized as a corporation).

*Authorization.* Is creditor's or lender's consent required to enter agreements or transfer assets?

*Assurance/good standing letter.* Full disclosure from attorneys, accountants, and malpractice insurers.

*Financial statements.*
  Audited balance sheet statements for the preceding 4 years.
  List of all long- and short-term debt.
  Financial covenants, with maturity dates.
  List of all accounts receivable, accounts payable, depreciation, and liabilities.

*Tax returns for the preceding 4 years.* Federal, state, and local; unusual correspondence or information.

*List of employees and insurance plans accepted.*
  Restrictive covenant agreements.
  Fringe benefits, insurances offered.

*Involvement in litigation.* Pleadings, insurance coverage.

*Material contracts/commitments.*
  Loans/lease and credit agreements.
  Sale/purchase of businesses.
  Management, third-party, and managed care contracts.

*Licenses/permits, agency filings.*

*Property owned.*
  Mortgages of tangible assets.
  Liens and security interests.

---

recent profit and loss statement; a list of short- and long-term debt with maturity dates; the amount of accounts receivable and accounts payable; depreciation schedules; and assumed liabilities. Are there any local property taxes due that follow the purchaser? Has any unusual legal or financial correspondence been recently received by the seller?

What are the details of the present staff members' terms of employment and fringe benefit plans? Is the restrictive covenant, noncompete clause, or liquidated damages reasonable? What material contracts, commitments, leases, and consignments are the practice obligated to fulfill? Obtain copies and evaluate all management, third-party, and managed care contracts. Ascertain what licenses or permits are required to operate the business. Are any types of agency filings necessary? Obtain copies of any tangible property liens, liabilities, chattel mortgages, security interests, and Uniform Commercial Code filings that the purchaser will assume.

The sequence of transferring practice ownership is shown in Figure 11–1. Both buyer and seller independently create their own goals and each has different sets of required resources. However, the goals must be compatible for the eventual completion of the sale. A detailed list of all the other events of a practice transfer is shown in Table 11–2 and requires the participation and cooperation of all concerned parties.

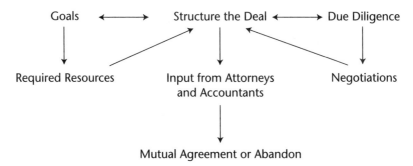

**Figure 11–1 Sequence of events for the transfer of ownership: The major participants and actions that must be taken to complete a transfer.**

**Table 11–2   Significant Events in Practice Transfer**

1. Buyer-seller interviews.
2. Confirmation of purchaser.
3. Independent appraisal.
4. Negotiation and compromise.
5. Agreement to terms, including restrictive covenant.
6. Offer to purchase signed and earnest money placed in escrow (optional step, parties may directly negotiate terms of purchase and sale agreement).
7. Financing, if required, sought.
8. Contracts, leases, profit and loss statements, tax returns, provider agreements, assets, and inventory verified.
9. Purchase and sales agreement signed.
10. Total value apportioned among various assets for IRS Form 8594 tax declaration.
11. Payoff or transfer of liabilities.
12. Title transferred.
13. Vendors and suppliers notified.
14. Third-party and managed care plan credentials applied for.
15. Patients notified.

## Valuation Methods

The basis for analyzing the value of a business can be found in Revenue Ruling 59-60 of the Internal Revenue Service (IRS). A summary of the main sections shows the following should be included as part of any appraisal:

1. Legal status of the business—information about the practitioner and the practice.
2. How similar practices sold recently compare in price to the practice under consideration. How the local and national economy affect the practice.
3. Book value adjustment of the balance sheet and a profit and loss statement should be performed to reflect the present fair market value of the depreciated tangible assets.

4. A valuation that takes into account both income and excess profits (if any) using capitalization rate methodology should be performed.
5. Goodwill, records, and restrictive covenants that are the intangible components of a practice should be examined carefully and assigned reasonable values as a result of thorough analysis.

The fair market value of a practice, as defined by Internal Revenue Service Ruling 59-60 and the American Society of Appraisers, is "the amount at which a practice would change hands between a willing buyer and a willing seller, each having reasonable knowledge of all the pertinent facts and market conditions, neither being compelled nor obligated to buy or sell, and with an exchange of equal consideration to both parties."[3] Another part of Internal Revenue Service Ruling 59-60 elaborates on what additional factors, both external in the marketplace and internal to the practice, have an impact on final value. These factors, once identified, should be taken into consideration:

1. The nature and history of the enterprise from its inception.
2. The economic outlook in general and the industry in particular.
3. The financial condition and earning capacity of the enterprise.
4. Identify the existence of goodwill or other intangible value, if relevant.
5. The market price of similar enterprises having traded in a free and open market.

No set formula or rule-of-thumb method can be applied to simplify the fair market valuation process. For this reason, a weighted average of several methods is suggested to estimate fair market value. Revenue Ruling 59-60 states that "a sound valuation will be based on all relevant facts, but the elements of common sense, informed judgment and reasonableness must enter into the process of weighing those facts and determining their aggregate significance." An appraiser may choose among several acceptable methods when determining the fair market value of a practice. The methods can be divided into three basic categories: asset approaches, income approaches, or market approaches.

The asset-based approach values the two primary components that contribute to practice value: tangible assets and intangible assets. Tangible assets include equipment, machinery, instruments, furnishings, leasehold improvements, supplies, and inventory. The methods used to value tangible assets are either fair market value (using comparable sales data and price listings of used equipment) or the "book value" remaining from the original depreciation basis obtained from the seller's tax returns. Current and unused inventory are valued using this method or simply the wholesale replacement cost. Intangible assets include goodwill, lease value, telephone number, practice name, income producing ability, and quality of patient records—all factors that should help minimize patient attrition during and after the transition.

The income approach develops a value for the practice using a viewpoint similar to what an investor might take when considering the purchase of a business with comparable investment characteristics. The calculations involved in this method determine that the value of a practice today is equal to what the practice can generate in the future for the new owner. This is determined by adding the future annual net cash flow of the business for a designated number of years. This total is then "discounted" back to present day using a present value formula that will be explained later in this chapter. The "discount rate" is equivalent to the estimated rate of return on the investment in the practice, and its value is reflected in the inherent risk of the purchase.

The market approach takes into account the significant benchmark variables of the practice, such as net-to-gross ratio, percent of staff salaries, cost of goods sold, and overhead, then compares these numbers to previous sales of similar practices. Once this analysis is completed, a guideline ratio as a percentage of past year's gross revenue is calculated to determine practice value. Unfortunately, information about sales of similar practices is difficult to obtain because it is used primarily for proprietary purposes by commercial brokers and research houses. Possible sources of comparative practice sales data are the Goodwill Registry in Plymouth Meeting, Pennsylvania; the Institute of Business Appraisers in Boynton Beach, Florida; and private ophthalmic appraisers found through the national organizations.

## Goodwill

Goodwill comprises the reputations of both the practice (professional) and practitioner (personal). Due to its controversial nature encompassing a variety of meanings, goodwill is the most complicated component of practice value to measure. A comprehensive examination of professional goodwill is beyond the scope of this text, but a brief discussion is relevant to an understanding of how goodwill, at times referred to as the *blue sky* portion of practice value, influences value.[4] One definition of *goodwill* established by the court system is

> property of an intangible nature constituting a valuable asset of the business of which it is part . . . Often a large portion of intrinsic marketable or assessable value of a business consists of its goodwill. However, goodwill could not be separated from the business from which it inheres, nor can it be disposed of independently from the business. It has no existence as property in and of itself as a separate and extinct identity, but only as incident of a continuing business having locality of name.[5]

A different court ruling defined *goodwill* as "the favor or advantage in the way of custom that a business has acquired in earning power beyond a mere value of its tangible assets."[2] This would imply that any amount paid beyond the fair market value of the practice's tangible assets is considered payment for goodwill. One definition of *goodwill* generally accepted by the accounting profession is "expectations of future profits under the ownership of someone other than the present owner."[4] This is supported by another definition, resulting from litigation: "goodwill is the favor which the management of a business has won from the public, and probability that old customers will continue their patronage."[6] Both of these suggest the likelihood that expected or future earnings should have an influence on the present value of a practice. The asset-based approach using the excess earnings method of practice valuation takes into account both definitions of *goodwill*.

In the eyes of the IRS,

goodwill is based upon earning capacity . . . and its value, therefore rests upon the excess of net earnings over and above a fair return on net tangible assets . . . such factors as prestige and renown of the business, the ownership of a trade or brand name and a record of successful operation over a prolonged period of time in a particular locality, also may furnish a report for inclusion in tangible value.[7]

The practice characteristics identified in Table 11–3 may contribute in some degree to determining the ultimate worth of goodwill. The value of goodwill can range from "an amount equal to your gross for the most recent four months to one-fourth of the preceding year's net."[8] This figure, in many cases, can encompass a wide range of value, adding to the dilemma inherent in the valuation of goodwill. This lends support to the argument that a practice must be valued using several different methods to properly assess the contribution of goodwill to total practice value.

## Business Risk Analysis

The capitalization rate is a numeric value derived to approximate the risk associated with continuation of the cash flow of the practice. The capitalization rate is "any divisor (usually expressed as a percentage) used to convert income into value." Capitalizing, therefore, is a "process that converts a single flow of economic income into an indication of value."[9] Expressed as a percentage, the more stable the business income stream, the lower the capitalization rate; and in turn, the more uncertain the business income stream, the higher the capitalization rate. This range or difference in values is considered the risk inherent in the future earning potential or cash flow stream of the practice, or the asset value in this case. The capitalization rate can be determined by a variety of methods, but one popular way is the "build-up method" of comparable return rates for various levels of cash flow risks. The starting point is the risk-free rate, which is equivalent to the long-term U.S. Treasury bond market yield. The next level of risk is reflected by the long-horizon expected equity risk premium

**Table 11-3    Practice Parameters That Influence Goodwill**

1. Gross income trend of preceding 3 years.
2. Net/gross ratio of preceding 3 years.
3. Location.
4. Competition.
5. Recall effectiveness.
6. Patient profile and fee structure.
7. Staff efficiency.
8. Lease terms.
9. Number of hours worked per week.
10. Number of weeks worked per year.
11. Whether practice is operating at full capacity or resources are underutilized.
12. Whether practice is a turnkey operation or in need of extensive renovation and equipment update.
13. The demographics of the local drawing area.
14. The new-to-former-patient ratios and rate of retention.
15. How current and advanced are the management information systems.
16. Similarity between the seller's and buyer's personalities and chairside styles.
17. The seller's reputation within the community and among colleagues.
18. The quality, legibility, and completeness of the patient records.
19. Whether practice is known in the community for providing any specialty services.
20. The projected annual growth potential.
21. Longevity of employee retention.
22. Active marketing and public relations programs.
23. Priority and budgetary allocations given to marketing records.

found in common stock. Added to this is a risk premium for the size of the business, in this case equivalent to the expected small stock risk premium, and finally, a subjective assessment of the risk premium for the lack of liquidity or salability of the specific business under consideration.

The sum of all the previously mentioned risk premiums will yield the total adjusted discount rate used in the discounted cash flow method of calculating value for the practice under consideration. The discount rate is "a rate of return used to convert a monetary sum (or series of monetary sums), payable or receivable in the future, into present value."[9] To determine the capitalization rate, the projected annual growth as a percentage for future practice revenue is deducted from the discount rate. Table 11–4 shows how to determine the final capitalization rate by using the build-up method. The first three values are taken from Ibbotson Associates, *Stocks, Bonds, Bills and Inflation Yearbook* (SBBI).[10] The last figure, the subjective business risk premium, is determined by the appraiser. Table 11–5 is an informal guide to

**Table 11–4    Build-up Method of Discount Rate Determination**

| | |
|---|---|
| Risk-free long-term 20-year Treasury bond | 6.7% |
| Long-horizon, large-cap stock risk premium | 7.5% |
| Expected small-cap stock size premium | 3.5% |
| Subjective business risk premium including | |
|     Industry barriers to entry, managed care | 1.5% |
|     Management depth and competence | 0.5% |
|     Practice, specific degree of diversification | 1.0% |
|     Dependence on key person | 1.5% |
|     Local barriers to entry | 1.0% |
|     Trends: sales growth, margins, net income | 0.5% |
| **Discount rate (total)** | **23.7%** |
| Less: Projected annual growth | 4.0% |
| **Capitalization rate (total)** | **19.7%** |

**Table 11–5    Qualitative Assessment to Choose a Discount Rate**

| *Description* | *Discount Rate* |
|---|---|
| Extremely stable | .16 |
| Very stable | .19 |
| Stable | .22 |
| Moderately stable | .25 |
| Questionable | .28 |
| Moderately unstable | .31 |

use when choosing a capitalization rate based on your qualitative judgment of the risks inherent in the continuing ability of the practice to earn income. The capitalization rate is then applied to the value of excess earnings to estimate the value of practice goodwill and other intangible assets.

## Excess Earnings Formula Method

Excess earnings are the earnings attributable to goodwill and other intangible assets, as opposed to tangible assets. The excess earnings method originates from the U.S. Treasury Department Appeals and Review Memorandum (ARM) 34, adopted to determine the goodwill of a business. In 1968, the Internal Revenue Service replaced ARM 34 with IRS Ruling 68-609 (1968-2, C.B. 327), which still is in effect. Appendix 11–2 explains the steps to be followed when using one popular version of the excess earnings method. This method, sometimes referred to as the *formula method*, often is associated with the following remarks:

> Goodwill can be thought of as the difference between an established successful business and one that has yet to establish itself and achieve success. The price the buyer should be willing to pay depends on the earning power and potential of the business. The price the seller should be content with is the amount considered as compensation for the transfer of intangible values and the surrender of the expected earning power of the business. The seller should base the value of goodwill on the actual condition and earning power of the business.[11]

Applying the excess earnings "formula" method to the numbers in a sample practice with financial characteristics as in Table 11–6 should clarify some of the more difficult steps to follow. One version for determining practice value using the excess earnings method is as follows:[12]

*Step 1.* Determine the adjusted net fair market value of the tangible assets. In this case, we use the book value of the fixed assets from the balance sheet plus the inventory. From this, we deduct any liabilities associated with the assets: in this case, half

## Table 11–6   Select Data from Income and Expense Statement

| | |
|---|---|
| Gross revenue | $450,000 |
| Cost of goods sold (28%) | $126,000 |
| Rent (8%) | $36,000 |
| Advertising (3%) | $13,500 |
| Insurance (2%) | $9,000 |
| Depreciation (4%) | $18,000 |
| Staff salaries (18%) | $81,000 |
| Phone, utilities (3%) | $13,500 |
| ECP's pension (1%) | $4,500 |
| Other expenses (4%) | $18,000 |
| Dues, magazines (1%) | $4,500 |
| Continuing education, meals (1%) | $4,500 |
| Pretax profit (29%) | $130,500 |
| Total effective tax (26%) | $33,930 |
| Working capital | $45,000 |
| *Abbreviated balance sheet data:* | |
| Cash (3%) | $13,500 |
| Accounts receivable (5%) | $22,500 |
| Inventory (8%) | $36,000 |
| *Total current assets* | $72,000 |
| Fixed assets (22%)* | $99,000 |
| *Total assets* | $171,000 |
| Accounts payable (4%) | $18,000 |
| Notes payable (2%) | $9,000 |
| *Total current liabilities* | $27,000 |
| Long-term debt (9%) | $40,500 |
| Net worth (23%) | $103,500 |
| *Total liabilities and net worth* | $171,000 |

*While this calculation typically uses book value, a more useful figure may result from using appraised fair market value, especially if there is a significant difference between book and fair market value.

the long-term debt of $40,500 used to previously purchase equipment. (Short-term debt is deducted in full.)

| | |
|---|---|
| Fixed assets | $99,000 |
| Inventory | $36,000 |
| Subtotal | $135,000 |
| Less liabilities | ($20,250) |
| Total | $114,750 |

*Step 2.* Estimate annual earning potential of the adjusted net tangible assets (step 1). To do this, multiply the tangible asset value by an interest rate 2 points higher than the cost of borrowed funds. In this case, add 2 percentage points to a 7% bank loan rate:

$$\$114{,}750 \times 0.09 = \$10{,}328,$$

this is the earning potential of tangible assets if an equivalent amount of money were invested.

*Step 3.* Ascertain the average annual income of an ECP in the area. Obtaining this information from either the most recent AOA Economic Surveys or the state's Bureau of Labor Statistics shows a figure of $105,000.

*Step 4.* Determine the annual net earnings of the business by adding the owner's adjusted salary and the practice's net profit (both before taxes). Include depreciation and other personal benefits taken as an expense. Normally, this can be an averaged or a weighted average taken of the most recent 2–4 years, but in this case, we simply use the 1 year figures in the sample data.

| | |
|---|---|
| Depreciation | $18,000 |
| ECP's pension | $4,500 |
| CE, meals | $4,500 |
| Pretax profit | $130,500 |
| Total | $157,500 |

*Step 5.* Determine the excess earning power by subtracting steps 2 and 3 from step 4:

$$\$157{,}500 - \$10{,}328 - \$105{,}000 = \$42{,}172,$$

this is the excess earnings or the amount of earnings above a fair return on the net tangible asset value.

*Step 6.* Determine the value of the practice's intangible assets by choosing an appropriate capitalization rate (figured previously from the build-up method in the discussion under business risk) to apply to the excess earnings (step 5):

$$\$42,172/0.197 = \$214,071.$$

*Step 7.* Determine the practice value by adding the tangible assets (step 1) and the value of the intangible assets (step 6):

$$\$214,071 + \$114,750 = \$328,821,$$

this is the indicated practice value as determined by the excess earnings method. Although this method may appear simple, it is relied on quite frequently. However, this value alone is not the final value but is used as part of a weighted average in combination with the values obtained from the next two methods.

## Discounted Cash Flow Method

The second method, the discounted cash flow (DCF) method, offers a valuation based on future earning capacity and recent financial performance. It takes into account gross revenue, practice operating expenses, depreciation, local-area going-rate ECP compensation, liabilities, and inflation. The DCF model offers the user an analysis similar to that performed by chief financial officers to make investment decisions. This requires the use of a spreadsheet that projects future revenue and expenses based on recent annual changes in practice performance and expected changes in variables that could affect future outcomes. The method can also factor in anticipated changes in operation, such as allocating less revenue to income or more to wages. A discount rate, which is the rate of return based on the inherent risk the business reflects, is applied to the sum of future cash flows to calculate the effective value of the practice in terms of present-day dollars. The theory behind the discounted future cash flow method is that the present value of a business entity is worth its expected future earnings. The discount rate, which accounts for the overall stability of the practice to continue producing cash flow and to retain the patient base, is determined from the build-up method previously demonstrated.

Many factors affecting practice value are intangible, such as goodwill and records, and so their worth is inherently arguable. *Goodwill*, in this context, is defined as the likelihood a business will continue operating under new ownership. In the past, transition to a new owner would be considered more secure the longer the seller was willing to stay on and "transfer" his or her patient loyalty to the "protégé." In the new world of managed health care economics, what is the seller's rapport with his patients worth to a buyer if 85% of the patients are enrolled in various managed care vision plans that may be closed to new providers and not transferable from the selling practitioner? Why would a purchaser want to buy a practice if a good possibility exists that the majority of the plan's members will pursue other directions for vision care? This recent development has become a factor for consideration when valuing practices in today's marketplace.

The subjectivity associated with the valuation of major intangible factors is a chronic problem in determining practice value. The valuation of goodwill must be considered very cautiously. In most instances, it is wiser to emphasize projected revenues and expenses, which is why the discounted cash flow method has become quite popular in the past decade. The concept of the present value of money is fundamental to an understanding of this method, because it uses basic business principles to make comparisons of different business opportunities based on the projected income and expenses.

## Present Value

What is $1,000 worth at 10%, tax deferred, in 1, 2, and 3 years? This is simply an example of compounding obtained by multiplying the interest received by the accrued principal for a specified number of years, the formula for which is

$$FV = PV \times (1 + r)^t$$

where FV = future value; PV = present value; $r$ = interest rate in decimals; and $t$ = number of compounding periods (years).

If we put this on a timeline, where 0 is the first day, 1 is the end of the first full year, 2 is the end of the second full year, and so on, the schematic of the interest received is

| Time in years | 0 | 1 | 2 | 3 |
|---|---|---|---|---|
| Cash flow | (1,000) | 100 | 110 | 121 + 1,000 (principal return) |

By convention, any money invested or spent is written with a negative symbol or in parentheses; therefore, on the first day, or 0 on the timeline, there is a negative $1,000. After that, at the end of each year, only the cash flow from the investment or interest received is written. At the end of the first compounding year the interest received is

$$\$1,000\,(0.10) = \$100,$$

this is the interest earned at the end of year 1.

Adding the interest received after year 1 to the initial principal gives the new principal amount for the second compounding year:

$$\$1,100\,(0.10) = \$110,$$

this is the interest earned at the end of year 2.

Adding the interest received after year 2 to the cumulative first 2-year principal gives the new principal amount for the third compounding year:

$$\$1,210\,(0.10) = \$121,$$

this is the interest earned at the end of year 3.

At the end of year 3, you receive your initial principal plus the 3 years' accrued interest, $1,331 total, which is the 3 years' compounding total.

Now, reverse the process. What is the present value of $1,331 received 3 years from today? This is an example of discounting, the formula for which is

$$PV = FV/(1 + r)^t = \$1,331/(1.10)^3.$$

For time in years = 0, 1, 2, and 3,

$$\$1{,}000 \leftarrow \underline{\qquad} \ \$1{,}331/(1.10)^3.$$

What is the value in 1 year of $1,331 received 3 years from today?

$$\$1{,}100 \leftarrow \underline{\qquad} \ \$1{,}331/(1.10)^2.$$

What is the value in 2 years of $1,331 received 3 years from today?

$$\$1{,}210 \leftarrow \$1{,}331/(1.10)^1.$$

Net Present Value = – (Initial Cost) + $\Sigma$ Cash Flows$/(1 + r)^t$,

where $r$ = the discount rate or cost of borrowed funds and should reflect the risk involved and $t$ = the number of years or compounding/discounting periods.

Appendix 11–3 offers a simple exercise to perform using the present value concept. The answer is found in Appendix 11–4.

Returning to the example of the practice sale, once the adjusted cash flows for the practice are determined and projected, present value is calculated to determine the current worth of the practice, using the discount rate that most closely reflects the risks inherent in those future cash flows. A step-by-step description of the discounted cash flow method using net present value calculations and the previous sample practice data follows.

## Determining Practice Value Using Discounted Cash Flow

Appendix 11–5 explains the steps that are performed during the discounted cash flow method. Refer to the spreadsheet shown in Table 11–7 and apply its sample practice parameters to complete the steps to calculate the discounted cash flow as follows.

*Step 1.* List gross revenue as $450,000 and for years 2–5 remember that the sample practice has an estimated annual growth rate of 4%.

**Table 11–7  Spreadsheet for Present Value of Discounted Cash Flows Method**

| Year | 1 | 2 | 3 | 4 | Terminal |
|---|---|---|---|---|---|
| Revenue | $450,000 | $468,000 | $486,720 | $506,188.8 | $526,436.352 |
| Operating expenses | ($292,500) | ($301,275) | ($310,313) | ($319,623) | ($329,211) |
| Depreciation | ($18,000) | ($18,000) | ($18,000) | ($18,000) | ($18,000) |
| OD substitute salary | ($105,000) | ($109,200) | ($113,568) | ($118,111) | ($122,835) |
| Pretax income | $34,500 | $39,525 | $44,839 | $50,455 | $56,390 |
| Effective tax (26%) | ($8,970.00) | ($10,276.50) | ($11,658.08) | ($13,118.41) | ($14,661.37) |
| Posttax income | $25,530 | $29,249 | $33,181 | $37,337 | $41,729 |
| Add back depreciation | $18,000 | $18,000 | $18,000 | $18,000 | $18,000 |
| Liabilities | ($8,100) | ($8,100) | ($8,100) | ($8,100) | ($8,100) |
| Net cash flow | $35,430 | $39,149 | $43,081 | $47,237 | $51,629 |

Present value at rate of 23.7% = $232,119.
Gross revenue = $450,000.
Adjusted operating expenses (total expenses − depreciation − personal benefit [taken as expense + COGS]) = $292,500.
Effective tax bracket = 26%.
Discount rate = 0.237 (previously calculated, see Business Risk Analysis).
Financing period = 4 yrs. + capitalized terminal year.
Income (substitute employment salary) = $105,000.
Depreciation = $18,000 per year for five years.
Liabilities = long-term debt (debt due longer than present fiscal year) divided into 5 equal years.

286

*Step 2.* Deduct the total adjusted operating expenses of $292,500 from the gross revenue. For years 2–5, assume the practice's operating expenses will increase by 3% each year.

*Step 3.* Deduct depreciation (the amount deducted from the gross revenue to recapture the purchase price of practice assets) of $18,000 per year to maintain current investment in equipment.

*Step 4.* Determine pretax income by subtracting $105,000, the normalized income an employed ECP would receive in the practice with 4% annual increases.

*Step 5.* Calculate the tax due by multiplying step 4 by the effective tax bracket of 26%.

*Step 6.* Determine posttax income by subtracting step 5 from pretax income.

*Step 7.* Add back depreciation.

*Step 8.* Deduct total liabilities amortized on a straight-line 5-year basis. This will yield the net cash flow for that year.

*Step 9.* Calculate the present value. The fair market value of any ongoing business is the present worth of the future cash flows, as shown in the PV formula, where $r$ is the discount rate and $C$ is the capitalization rate that equals the discount rate less the projected annual growth:

$$\text{Present Value} = \sum (\text{Future Year Cash Flows})/(1 + r) \\ + (\text{Terminal Year Cash Flow}/C)/(1 + r)$$

Don't forget to capitalize the last year before you discount all the cash flows.

$$PV = CF1/(1 + r)^1 + CF2/(1 + r)^2 + CF3/(1 + r)^3 \\ + CF4/(1 + r)^4 + (CF5/C)/(1 + r)^5$$

$$PV = 35{,}430/(1.237)^1 + 39{,}149/(1.237)^2 + 43{,}081/(1.237)^3$$
$$+ 47{,}237/(1.237)^4 + (51{,}629/0.197)/(1.237)^5,$$

where PV = present value; CF = net cash flow; $r$ = discount rate; and C = capitalization rate.

Table 11–7 shows the spreadsheet application to determine the present value for the sample practice. Determining the capitalization rate as 19.7% and the discount rate as 23.7% for 5 years indicates a value of $232,119.

## Market Comparison Approach—Gross Revenue Multiplier Method

In the third valuation approach, the gross revenue multiplier method, the appraiser looks at two areas: the practice's performance compared to national medians and data from the sale of similar practices. Based on subjective judgment of how the practice fares in these areas, a percentage multiplier is applied to the past year's gross revenue, giving an indication of value. The process of determining value based on a comparative judgment follows.

*Step 1.* Obtain statistics similar to the data found in Table 11–8 for comparison. The appraiser knows the range that most practices sell for relative to gross revenue and takes this into account when comparing the practice being appraised to similar ones that have sold.

*Step 2.* Next, the appraiser would compare the practice's performance in several areas to established norms, such as those in the AOA's 1998 Caring for the Eyes of America Survey or median figures found in Robert Morris Associates Industry Statistics:

| Variable | Sample Practice | Median | Comparison |
|---|---|---|---|
| Net/Gross | 29.0% | 31.0% | – |
| COGS | 28.0% | 28.0% | = |
| Pension | 1.0% | 1.8% | – |
| Employee wages | 18.0% | 15.3% | – |
| Other expenses | 4.0% | 10.8% | + |
| Rent, utilities, phone | 11.0% | 6.7% | – |
| Insurance | 2.0% | 1.3% | – |
| Depreciation | 4.0% | 2.4% | + |

*Step 3.* The appraiser notes that the practice's performance ranks above national medians in two areas and below national medians in five others. Based on that information and the appraiser's judgment of how the practice compares to those previously sold, a multiplier is assigned subjectively. In the sample practice, a 0.55 multiplier is chosen.

*Step 4.* To determine practice value, apply the multiplier to the practice's past year gross revenue:

$$0.60 \times \$450{,}000 = \$270{,}000$$

## Determining Final Practice Value

Final practice value is determined by using a weighted average of the three appraisal methods. Because the excess earnings approach requires the fewest assumptions, this method is given the most weight. Conversely, the least weight is placed on the discounted cash flow method, which requires the most assumptions about future performance. Assign an average weight to the market gross revenue multiplier, which is based on comparison to actual sales and other appraisals.

*Step 1.* To review, we came up with the following values using each method:

| | |
|---|---|
| Excess earnings | $328,821 |
| Discounted cash flow | $232,119 |
| Market gross revenue multiplier | $270,000 |

**Table 11–8    Recent Practice Sales Data (listed in order of gross revenue)**

| State | Year | Gross Revenue | Adjusted Net Revenue | Sale Price* | Tangible Assets | Ratio of Sale Price/ Gross Revenue |
|---|---|---|---|---|---|---|
| Massachusetts | 1999 | 1,009 | 286 | 450 | 103 | 45% |
| Florida | 2000 | 971 | 231 | 622 | 101 | 64% |
| New Hampshire | 1999 | 920 | 185 | 535 | 149 | 58% |
| Connecticut | 1998 | 902 | 278 | 508 | 113 | 56% |
| New Jersey | 1999 | 834 | 258 | 514 | 99 | 61% |
| Texas | 1998 | 752 | 175 | 500 | 116 | 68% |
| Michigan | 1996 | 725 | NA | 218 | 102 | 30% |
| Pennsylvania | 1999 | 621 | 98 | 360 | 88 | 58% |
| South Carolina | 1999 | 579 | 161 | 350 | 97 | 60% |
| Maine | 1997 | 558 | 196 | 400 | 85 | 71% |
| Virginia | 1995 | 550 | NA | 275 | 275 | 50% |
| Texas | 1999 | 488 | 80 | 130 | 72 | 27% |
| New Jersey | 2000 | 468 | 96 | 200 | 68 | 43% |
| Massachusetts | 1997 | 440 | 120 | 190 | NA | 43% |
| Rhode Island | 1996 | 424 | 101 | 209 | 82 | 49% |
| Connecticut | 1999 | 366 | 111 | 205 | 35 | 56% |
| Vermont | 1999 | 328 | 95 | 175 | NA | 53% |
| New York | 1996 | 307 | 57 | 150 | 79 | 49% |
| Connecticut | 1997 | 276 | 85 | 175 | 65 | 64% |
| Florida | 1998 | 259 | 31 | 105 | 52 | 41% |
| Pennsylvania | 1999 | 230 | 82 | 103 | 88 | 45% |
| Massachusetts | 1997 | 204 | 65 | 61 | 35 | 30% |
| Connecticut | 1997 | 202 | 54 | 98 | 47 | 49% |
| Massachusetts | 1998 | 177 | 42 | 55 | 24 | 31% |
| Massachusetts | 1995 | 128 | 36 | 48 | 18 | 38% |

*In some cases appraised price where transfer is pending or under consideration.

*Step 2.* Assign each value the appropriate weight.

| | |
|---|---|
| Excess earnings | $328,821 × 3 = $986,463 |
| Discounted cash flow | $232,119 × 1 = $232,119 |
| Market gross revenue multiplier | $270,000 × 2 = $540,000 |

*Step 3.* To come up with the weighted average, which is the final practice value, add the weighted figures and divide by 6:

$$\$1,758,582/6 = \$293,097$$

This is the final practice value.

## Breakeven Point Analysis

Breakeven point analysis will not determine the value of a practice or for what price a practice should sell. However, it offers a method of calculating the feasibility of affording the monthly payments based on current practice revenues and expenses, projected financial performance, desired personal salary, and contracted selling price. An example of how to calculate this follows. We use the sample practice that grosses $450,000 per year, whose sale price is $290,000, of which $250,000 is financed for 10 years at 9% interest.

*Step 1.* Average gross monthly income for this practice is $450,000/12 = $37,500.

*Step 2.* Determine the total fixed expenses (TFE), which include salary, rent, insurance, utilities, and so forth; for this example, 40% of gross income will be used as the TFE ($180,000 annually or $15,000 average per month).

*Step 3.* Determine monthly payments for the loan of $3,167. This is obtained from an amortization schedule.

*Step 4.* Determine desired practitioner income, for which we will use $90,000 annually or $7,500 per month.

*Step 5.* Determine total fixed cost (TFC), which equals the sum of total fixed expenses, debt service payments, and practitioner income:

$$TFC = TFE + \text{debt service} + ECP \text{ income}$$

In this case the total of the three figures is $25,667, based on a monthly average.

*Step 6.* The formula for breakeven point (BEP)

$$BEP = TFC/(1 - VC \text{ [in \%]})$$

VC = variable costs: lab bills or the cost of goods sold (COGS), which is 28% in this example.

$$BEP = \$25,667/(1.0 - 0.28) = \$25,667/0.72 = \$35,649.$$

Since this is less than the average total monthly revenue of $37,500 by $1,851, there is enough income to make the desired salary plus pay off the debt and operate the practice with the present revenues and expenses. There is a cushion or safety factor of $1,851 per month or $22,212 annually in this example. If the breakeven point is higher than the monthly revenue of $37,500 then the options are these: (1) take less income, (2) reduce monthly debt service payments by choosing a longer loan repayment schedule, (3) reduce the amount of the monthly total fixed expenses (difficult to do), or (4) decline the purchase.

## Degree of Difficulty in Valuing Practice Assets and Liabilities

Part of the difficulty in assigning a value to a practice depends on the practice's assets and liabilities.

Tangible assets:

| | |
|---|---|
| Equipment | not difficult |
| Inventory | easy |
| Office lease premium | difficult |
| Leasehold improvements | moderately difficult |
| Accounts receivable | slightly difficult |

Intangible assets:

| | |
|---|---|
| Goodwill | very difficult |
| Records | moderately difficult |

Liabilities:

| | |
|---|---|
| Accounts payable | not difficult |
| Equipment leases due | not difficult |
| Office lease deficiencies | difficult |

It is worth mentioning that an intangible component of a practice often considered in practice valuation is how to assess the practice's growth potential. Although this certainly is a favorable intangible for the purchaser, it is uncertain and depends greatly on the new practitioner's efforts. Practice potential, as many sellers would hope, has yet to be realized and should not add significant cost to the purchaser, rather it can be promoted as an added incentive to buy a particular practice, if the buyer believes there is untapped income that can be realized.

Accounts receivable includes any money owed to the practice. The longer a patient's bill goes uncollected, the less likely it will ever be collected. Since these debts have been owed to the selling practitioner, there is little likelihood of a new person collecting them. For this reason, the new practitioner would be advised not to purchase the existing accounts receivable. But, if he or she does, the following is a guide to use when purchasing:

| *Age of Account Balance* | *Percent of Face Value to Pay* |
|---|---|
| >30 days | 60–80 |
| 30–60 days | 40–60 |
| 60–90 days | 20–40 |
| 90–120 days | 10–20 |
| 20+ days | 0 |

## Transfer of Records

Having an established patient base is the greatest advantage to purchasing an existing practice. In evaluating the practice, estimating the likelihood that patients will return is the most difficult unknown to assess. Patient records, in and of themselves, have no value. Possession of the patient record with name, address, telephone, and all prior eyecare data allows patients to feel that their care is being continued by the new practitioner and allows the new practitioner to internally market to an existing patient base. A healthy practice will have a 20–40% rate of new patient visits. This can be found by looking through patient records and determining the number of new patient visits over the last two years. Patients who were new to the practice prior to the last two years should have returned to the practice for subsequent care. This return rate also should be evaluated to determine how well the practice has been retaining patients.

Also, patient records should be sorted by the percentage of third party vs. private paying patients. Third-party patients will not generate the same gross revenue to the practice as private paying patients. Practices that have a large percentage of third-party patients need a larger patient base and can be transferred successfully only if the new practitioner can continue as a provider under the third-party plan. These patients generally have less loyalty to the selling practitioner than private patients. Their primary loyalty is to the office willing to provide them the same benefits.

Practices with a higher than average number of examinations but average gross income are either charging low fees or treating a large percentage of third-party patients. Records are a very difficult component to value for numerous reasons. The number of totally active patients is indeterminable; however, one method of estimation would be to consider all patients examined within the past 3 years as active and anyone who has not been examined in the office in 3 years can be considered inactive. Using an attrition factor, consider the number of active patients as

|  | *Percent of Active Patients* |
| --- | --- |
| Past year | 100% |
| 2 years | 75% (25% patient loss) |
| 3 years | 50% (50% patient loss) |
| Total | 225% |

Therefore, as an estimation technique, the total number of patients examined in the past 12 months times 2.25 will give the approximate number of total active patients. This total can be multiplied by $0.50–$4 per record, depending on quality of records, recall effectiveness, return rate of patients, age of patients, and dollar amounts spent by patients. The total of this gives an approximate value for the records alone. Records have tax-advantaged value to the buyer, therefore, they can be depreciated in cases where patient records can be shown to be a separate entity and have the following characteristics:[9]

1. An assignable value distinct from practice goodwill.
2. Goodwill alone did not determine repeat business.
3. Records have a limited useful life.
4. Records contain useful factual information for patient treatment.
5. The final purchase price was negotiated by an arm's-length agreement.

According to the American Medical Association, patients are not for sale nor are their records.[13] However, in the purchase and sale contract some mention should be made as to the buyer assuming "custody" of the seller's records. Also, to protect the buyer from any problems arising from possession of confidential patient records that person did not generate, the seller should notify all patients of their record transfer and that the record will now be with the purchasing ECP.[13] If, for any reason, the patient wants his or her records transferred elsewhere, this should be done upon written request by the patient (refer to Appendix 11–6, Sample Patient Record Transfer). If no written request is sent to the office, the buyer can assume the patient wishes that office to keep the record. The letter shown in Appendix 11–6 will serve the dual purpose of introducing the buyer into the practice and informing patients about the disposition of their records.

## Restrictive Covenant

In most cases, on entering into an employment situation with a senior ECP or purchasing a portion of a practice, the employment contract or purchase agreement will include what is known as a *restrictive covenant* or *covenant not to compete*. Simply put, this is an agreement that prevents either the selling party or a departing employee from competing for a specific period of time within a specified area. The intent being to prevent economic harm to the buyer or previous employer. This is an important protective principle that should be part of any purchase contract for a practice being assumed. Without this provision, the selling ECP would be free to open an office or work for someone else and possibly detract from the practice's goodwill by taking former patients to another location.

If the terms or limitations of the restrictive covenant are deemed to be unreasonable, and should it be challenged in court, it could be declared unenforceable. This is something to take into consideration when developing the elements included in any restrictive covenant. Four main components a restrictive covenant should include are time period, geographic area, mode of practice, and liquidated damages.[14] For a restrictive covenant to be considered valid by state courts, it should last only long enough to protect the purchaser from any possible harmful competition from the seller. This is determined by how often a patient comes to an ECP's office and how long it will take the new ECP to establish his or her own patient base. In general, restrictive covenants of up to 2 years have been upheld by the courts, while more than this has been successfully challenged as being unfair or not within the public favor.[15]

The second segment of the covenant, which concerns restriction on practicing within a specified geographic area, is accepted as reasonable if it prevents the seller from practicing in an area from which the practice normally obtains its patients.[16] The exact mileage will depend on the type of setting in which the practice is located. Therefore, a 5-mile restriction might be deemed unreasonable for a downtown urban practice but not necessarily for a rural setting. Restrictive covenants of up to 3 miles have been upheld, while more than this have been successfully challenged.

The third segment of the covenant, regarding type of activity, applies only to practices that would be likely to have a negative impact on or decrease the income of the practice that was sold.[17] Therefore, if the seller had an exclusive referral-only VT practice, it could be deemed unreasonable to prohibit him or her from fitting contact lenses but not from performing VT in a 3-mile radius for 2 years. And, finally, should the seller not honor the restrictive covenant, it would be wise to stipulate the amount (known as liquidated damages) to be paid if the need arises. This monetary award should be calculated to compensate for any projected damages or loss the practice might incur by competition from the departing practitioner's new endeavor. It is not an amount that should be used to punish or penalize, or it may be considered voidable.

In summary, as long as a restrictive covenant does not impinge on the public good, is not unjustly limiting, does not extend beyond an area that is essential to protect the buyer, is not unreasonable in its terms, and is no longer than 2 years or 3 miles, in most instances it will be found enforceable. One caution is that the restrictive covenant should not violate the Medicare antikickback statute, 42 U.S.C. Section 1320a-7b. In some cases, government officials have claimed that when practitioners "selling their practices continue to be affiliated with buyers of the practice, payments for intangibles (including covenants not to compete) could be considered disguised payments for future referrals."[18] To avoid this possibility, make sure the purchase price does not exceed fair market value.[19]

Finally, a tax benefit accrues to the buyer for the value of the restrictive covenant. The buyer can itemize and depreciate this amount over the life of the covenant. Therefore, the exact amount attributed to the restrictive covenant should be specified in the purchase agreement. It is in the buyer's best interest to include a reasonable covenant not to compete for his or her future protection.

## Ownership Transition

The time period during which the selling practitioner remains in the practice after the closing of the sale is known as the *transition period*. When handled properly, it should either add value for the seller or, at least, make the sale of the practice easier. The presence of the selling practitioner allows the purchaser to be introduced to the patients and build a level of familiarity with those patients who initially might be reluctant to see the newer practitioner. This generally translates into a higher retention rate. The longer the selling doctor remains in the practice, the higher is the percentage of existing patients who will probably be successfully transferred. During this time, the two practitioners have to work together, requiring a certain amount of compatibility. For the purchasing practitioner, it means accepting occasional objections in those cases where the patient has a very strong allegiance to the seller. For the selling practitioner, it means stepping back from control of the practice and fully support the new practitioner, especially with patients who might not easily accept change.

The transition period also allows the selling practitioner to introduce the new practitioner into the practice. This includes going over office procedures, ordering, suppliers, and working to transfer staff support. It means introducing the new practitioner to key people in the area, including the main referral sources of the practice.

The transition period applies to the staff as well. Having the existing staff remain in the office can be more valuable in some instances than having the selling practitioner remain. This is especially true when the staff member has been working in the office for many years and knows all the patients. Since the staff members are the first source of contact with the patients, both on the phone and in the office, they can be a vital link in easing any patient apprehension about seeing a new doctor.

The selling ECP should remain in the practice at least on a part-time basis for 4–6 months. Consider allowing the seller to examine patients 2 days per week for the first 2–3 months, then 1 day per week for the next 2–3-month period. This can be reduced to 1 day per week or every other week for an additional 3–6 months, at the discretion or need of the purchaser. If the seller is willing to stay on an additional year in an as-needed capacity, all the better. However, if the transfer time is less than 4 months, some allowance should be made for the buyer such as deducting a small (2–3) percentage of the price for each month less than the 4-month period. The purchasing doctor can expect to pay the selling practitioner for his or her time during the transition period. This usually is done on a fixed per diem or percentage of production basis. The new ECP may want to slightly increase the salaries of those staff people to be retained. This shows good faith on the part of the new practitioner and should pay for itself many times over in goodwill with every patient contact.

## Maximizing Practice Value

It is much easier to sell part of a practice to someone familiar with the practice rather than all of a practice to someone unfamiliar or a new buyer. Keeping these two "rules" in mind, the first obvious conclusion is to sell to an associate. If your goal is to maximize your return on investment, then plan well in advance; 5 years is not too early. Many established group practices have found this to be quite successful. The remaining ECP shareholding partners either buy the stock of the retiring ECP or the retiring ECP's ownership interest is replaced by a new associate-partner who purchases the shares. If you are in solo practice, it is in your best interest to plan ahead by taking on an associate for 1 or 2 years, even on a part-time basis, let this person buy a small ownership percentage interest in your practice, then 2–5 years after joining, let the associate purchase the remaining ownership interest while you ease out of active practice on your own schedule.

Analyze your financial picture, including profit margins (gross, operating, and net) and the past 3 years of trends and ratios. Make the declared net margin as high as possible during the 2 years prior to selling the practice by not taking extraordinary or excessive expenses. Remember, the buyer will use net income not gross income on which to base projections for living expenses and debt service payments. Improve the physical appearance and possibly update exam equipment. Have the required financial and practice analysis information readily available and in an easily understood format, including the last 3–5 years' tax returns and the most recent quarter's income and expense statement. Specific practice qualities that enhance value are a high percentage of patients over 65. This segment uses eye-care services far more than other groups and is eligible for Medicare. Capitation contracts with reasonable reimbursement levels are a source of guaranteed income that facilitates longer term planning. Managed care should probably be at a 50–70% penetration for an urban location, 35–55% for suburban, and 20–40% for rural. This source of income typically is less per unit output in your office, but the trend still is increasing, although at slower annual increments. Having the selling ECP remain with the practice on an as-needed, part-time basis for 2 years after the sale is beneficial. A location that is very visible, street level in a high traffic area, also is valuable. Finally, efficient operations that result in a net-to-gross ratio of 34% or better and adequately funded information technology and marketing budgets increase practice value, for which a buyer should be willing to pay.

An area that should be handled with caution includes valuing tangible assets at fair market value when allocating for tax purposes. Values that are inflated for depreciation benefit may be challenged if audited. Sales prices that are higher than 80% of the past year's gross revenues may be looked on as suspicious. To comply with antikickback regulations, it is recommended that seller financing be no longer than 1 year, because anything longer could be considered payment for steering patients to the practice. Both parties must include Form 8594 on the federal tax return for the year in which the sale takes place. The dollar amount for the allocation of value to all the tangible and intangible components must be the same for both the buyer and seller. It is recommended that tangibles not be overvalued or intangibles be undervalued.

## Tax Implications to Buyer and Seller

Since the most recent Tax Reform Act, the apportionment of dollar value to various parts of a practice transfer has become easy and less argumentative between the two involved parties. For the seller of a practice organized as a sole proprietorship, the tax implication can be reduced by allocating as much of the purchase price to those tangible assets that will be treated as long-term capital gain. Capital gain has a maximum federal tax of 20% compared to ordinary income of probably 33% or more. Consider

**Table 11–9    Tax Implications to Buyer and Seller**

| Assets | To Seller | To Buyer |
|---|---|---|
| 1. Equipment and furnishings | Potential depreciation recapture<br>Ordinary income | Step up in basis<br>5–10-year depreciation deduction |
| 2. Inventory and supplies | Ordinary income | Deducted when used |
| 3. Records and goodwill | Capital gain | 15-year amortization |
| 4. Restrictive covenant | Ordinary income over length of covenant | Deducted over length of covenant |

Information supplied by Alvin Levine, CPA, partner in the firm Rosenberg, Rich, Baker and Berman, Bridgewater, New Jersey, personal communication, October 12, 2000.

gifting your exam equipment to your children, if they are still young and your dependents, prior to the sale. In this event, the equipment is sold by your children at a much lower tax rate.[20] Allocate as much of the intangible value to goodwill and patient records, as these also qualify for long-term capital gain. For the seller, the covenant not to compete should have a minimum amount because this is taxed as ordinary income. One caution is to make sure that the allocation is completed as an *arm's-length agreement* with no hint of collusion, to minimize the tax implication, and that both the buyer and seller report the same values on IRS Form 8594. The present disposition of the various taxable assets of a practice sale is identified in Table 11–9.

## Action Plan for ECPs

1. Recognize the need to value the practice using at least three approaches: income, asset, and market comparison.
2. Decide when you believe it will be in your best interest to start the ownership transfer process.
3. Begin to assemble the information that will be required to complete an offer proposal.
4. Make those changes to the practice that will make it more desirable to prospective associates and maximize value.

# Proposal Information for Offer[2]

1. Brief history of the practice: age, location, and finances.
2. Tax returns for at least the past 3 years: for a sole proprietorship, Schedule C; for a partnership, Form 1065 and K-1; and for a professional service corporation, either Schedule 1120 or 1120S, if organized as a subchapter S corporation.
3. Profit and loss or income and expense statement and balance sheets, if available, for at least 3 years, but at least, the current year's quarterly statements.
4. Complete list of assets to be transferred by model, age, and fair market value.
5. Complete list of the wholesale or acquisition cost of the current, useable frame, spectacle, and contact lens inventory.
6. A map plotting the competition, using a radius of 1–2 miles in an urban area, 3–5 miles in a suburban area, and 7–10 miles in a rural area; differentiate optometrist, ophthalmologist, optician, and corporate chain.
7. A list of the current patient volume, using number of exams per year for the last 1–3 years and a breakdown of new and former patients by percentage in zip codes and age demographics, if available.
8. Fee schedules of all services and the percentage of specialty practice.
9. A sample of all practice promotional materials used.
10. A list of employees, their work schedules, and duties.
11. A list of all referral sources used.
12. Copies of all contracts, leases, and provider agreements.
13. Description of the community, including drawing area demographics.
14. A list of all insurance plans accepted.
15. Number of hours per week and number of weeks per year worked.

16. A sample sheet from the appointment book and a sample day sheet.
17. An explanation of how the asking price was determined.
18. A copy of the appraisal if available.
19. Description of what financing terms are being offered, if any.
20. A specification of how long the selling ECP is available for a transition period and on what basis.
21. Copies of any equipment and rental leases to be assumed by the purchaser.
22. A sample patient record.

# Popular Version of Excess Earnings Method[11]

*Step 1.* Determine the adjusted net fair market value of the tangible assets. This is best performed by a firm that specializes in equipment appraisals. If a fair market appraisal is not possible, the book value may be substituted but caution must be used, as a variance in final value may result. As a general rule, equipment and furnishings will depreciate about 20% per year from the original cost and stabilize at a "salvage" value between 20% and 30% of acquisition cost after 5 years. Inventory including current useable frames, spectacle lenses, and unopened contact lenses should be assigned a wholesale or replacement cost.

*Step 2.* Estimate the annual earning potential of the adjusted net tangible asset value (figure from step 1) in an alternate investment. Assume you had the equivalent amount of money instead of the equipment, furnishings, and inventory. If you placed this in a relatively safe investment, how much could you earn annually? Another way to figure equivalent earning potential is the rate of interest to borrow money? Both these probably would be 2–4 points higher than U.S. Treasury bonds.

*Step 3.* Ascertain the normal or median earnings of an ECP in the area. Another figure that can be used is the amount an ECP working as an employee operating the business would receive, but caution should be used as this can be artificially low. The going rate for an employed ECP can vary according to the area. The best sources to search for this data are the AOA Annual Economic Survey and your state's Bureau of Labor Statistics.

*Step 4.* Determine the adjusted annual net earnings of the business (net income before subtracting owner's salary and taxes). This should include all the personal benefits, both salary and fringe benefits, and personal items taken as expenses the owner receives.

*Step 5.* Determine the extra or excess earning power of the practice. Subtract the net earning power of the tangible assets (figure from step 2) plus reasonable substitute income of an ECP (figure from step 3) from the average net earnings (figure from step 4). The excess earnings are considered the amount of earnings above a fair return on the net tangible asset value.

*Step 6.* Determine the value of the intangible assets of the practice by choosing an appropriate capitalization rate to apply to the excess earnings, which are the earnings attributable to goodwill and other intangible assets, as opposed to tangible assets (step 1). This rate and the discount rate have been previously determined in the section on Business Risk.

*Step 7.* The final practice value is determined by adding the tangible asset value (figure from step 1) plus the goodwill and intangible asset value (figure from step 6).

# APPENDIX 11–3

# Determining Present Value

You saved $10,000 and now would like to earn a reasonable rate of return on an investment for 5 years. A safe mutual fund you are considering has averaged 8% total net interest, compounded annually, over the past 10 years and is expected to continue this performance. The present rate of return in a bank savings account is 4%. As an alternative, your friend Sneaky Pete wants a personal loan for his business expansion and has offered you the following two payback options for the initial $10,000:

|  | Option 1 | Option 2 |
|---|---|---|
| End of year 1 | 0 | $3,500 |
| End of year 2 | 0 | $3,500 |
| End of year 3 | 0 | $3,500 |
| End of year 4 | 0 | $3,500 |
| End of year 5 | $20,000 | $3,500 |

He is willing to pay you a $2,500 premium if he doesn't have to make yearly payments, which is reflected in the greater amount of payment in option 1. You assess the level of risk in Sneaky Pete's proposals to be 50% greater than the mutual fund option. If your goal is to maximize dollar return, which should you choose: option 1, option 2, or the mutual fund?

# Answers to Present Value Problem

| Year 0 | 1 | 2 | 3 | 4 | 5 |
|---|---|---|---|---|---|

Option 1

$(10,000) + 0/1.12^1 + \quad 0/1.12^2 + \quad 0/1.12^3 + \quad 0/1.12^4 + \quad 20,000/1.12^5$

Option 2

$(10,000) + 3,500/1.12^1 + 3,500/1.12^2 + 3,500/1.12^3 + 3,500/1.12^4 + 3,500/1.12^5$

Mutual Fund

$(10,000) + 800/1.08^1 + \quad 864/1.08^2 + \quad 933/1.08^3 + \quad 1,008/1.08^4 + 11,088/1.08^5$

After completing the three calculations, the net present values are as follows, which shows that option 2 would be the choice to maximize value:

NPV option 1 = $1,349
NPV option 2 = $2,617
NPV mutual fund = $509

# Discounted Cash Flow Method

Run through the following eight steps, using the spreadsheet data for years 1–5. Each set of calculations will give you the net cash flow for that year. The DCF process starts by listing gross revenue (line 1) and subtracting total adjusted operating costs, both fixed and variable (line 2) but not practitioner personal income; then subtracting depreciation (line 3) and subtracting the normalized income a substitute ECP would be paid in the practice (line 4) yields the pretax income (line 5). Multiply this number by the effective tax bracket to determine the tax due (line 6), subtract this amount from the pretax income to yield the posttax income (line 7). Add back depreciation (line 8) as a positive amount in order to determine net cash flow (line 9). Deduct or add any after tax expenses or credits (line 10), then total each vertical column to obtain adjusted cash flow (line 11). Finally, perform a present value calculation on the sum of all the cash flows choosing as a discount rate the business risk premium previously determined (line 12).

The present value is obtained using the following calculations:

*Step 1.* List *revenue* projected for a 5-year period with annual growth of +4.0%, using $450,000 as a base figure.

*Step 2.* Deduct *adjusted operating expenses* (total expenses – depreciation + COGS) projected for a 5-year period with annual growth of +3.0%.

*Step 3.* Deduct *depreciation* for a 5-year straight line period, using $18,000 per year as an average amount to keep current.

*Step 4.* Deduct *replacement ECP income* with a +4.0% annual increase.

*Step 5.* To calculate the *pretax income,* subtract steps 2–4 from step 1.

*Step 6.* Determine the *tax due,* using 26% as an effective tax bracket.

*Step 7.* Calculate the *posttax income* by subtracting step 6 from step 5.

*Step 8.* Add back the *depreciation.*

*Step 9.* Deduct any *liabilities* due on practice assets over a 5-year period.

*Step 10.* Add steps 7 and 8 less step 9 to yield the *adjusted net cash flow.*

*Step 11.* Determine the *discount rate* from build-up method. This is equal to the capitalization rate plus the projected annual growth.

*Step 12.* Calculate the *present value.*

# Sample Patient Record Transfer Letter

Dear _____:

This letter is to advise you that I am (*retiring from, selling*) my practice as of ____ (*MM/DD/YY*) ____. The reason for my departure is (*describe the reason here*). At this time, I would like to announce that Dr. _____ will be taking over my practice as of ____ (*MM/DD/YY*) ____ and will continue to provide the same high-quality eyecare you have received at this office for so many years. I believe Dr. _____'s ability and knowledge will satisfy your eyecare needs, and I personally instructed (*him, her*) in the important aspects that have made this practice unique and well appreciated by all of my patients.

Dr. _____ graduated from _____ optometry school and performed a postdoctorate residency at _____. I am very confident that you will quickly agree that I am leaving the practice in quite competent hands. In addition, the same loyal support staff with which you all are very familiar will be available to take care of your needs as well as answer any of your questions. Should you wish to make an appointment, simply call the same telephone number, _____. Our office hours will be _____.

A copy of your record will stay at this office; however, you are under no obligation to accept Dr. _____ as your primary eyecare practitioner. Should you desire to have your records transferred to another office, we need your written authorization and a completed record release form, which you can obtain by calling this office. If you wish to continue to use the services of this office, you may authorize the release of your records to Dr. _____ at your next visit.

In closing let me express my appreciation for your many years of loyalty, support and friendship. It has been a pleasure to be your optometrist. May I take this opportunity to wish you much happiness and good health in future years.

Respectfully,

## Notes

1. Tax court perspectives. *E-Law Business Valuation Perspective.* Mercer Capital Management newsletter. 1999;98(4).
2. Modified from Ginsberg A. *Financial Valuation of Your Practice.* Los Angeles: PMIC; 1991.
3. American Society of Appraisers. Definitions. *Business Valuation Standards.* Herndon, VA: American Society of Appraisers; 1994.
4. Determining the value of your practice. *Journal of the American Dental Association.* September 1984;109.
5. Buckl v. Buckl, 373 PA Super 521, 542 A. 2nd 65 (1988) (en banc).
6. Fexa v. Fexa, 578 PA A. 2nd 134 (PA Super 1990).
7. IRS Revenue Ruling 59-60.
8. Fallon K. What's your practice worth in cash? *Medical Economics.* January 22, 1979.
9. Pratt S, Reilly R, Schweihs R. *Valuing Small Businesses and Professional Practices.* New York: McGraw-Hill; 1998.
10. *Stocks, Bonds, Bills, and Inflation 1997.* Chicago: Ibbotson Associates; 1997:161.
11. Revenue Ruling 68-809, 1968-2, C.B. 327.
12. *How to Buy or Sell a Business,* Small Business Reporter Series. San Francisco: Bank of America; 1982.
13. American Medical Association. *Buying and Selling Medical Practices.* Chicago: AMA; 1990.
14. McNair R, Decator E. Medical practice acquisition: practical guidelines for the physician. *Medical Staff Counselor.* Winter 1990;1(4).
15. Westee Secretarial Service Inc. v. Westinghouse Elect. Corp.; 538 F. Suppl. 108 (E.D. PA 1982).
16. Beasley v. Banks; #873DC855 N.C. Count of App.; June 7, 1988.
17. Trilag Assoc. Inc. v. Famularo; 455 PA 243314A; 2nd 287; 1974.
18. Letter from D. McCarthy Thornton, general counsel to the Office of Inspector General, to T. Sullivan at the Internal Revenue Service, December 22, 1992.
19. Kurland R. Physician non-compete agreements must be carefully tailored. *Health Care News Letter.* April 1995;10(5):11–15.
20. Your gain may be a loss. *Dental Economics.* February 2000:136.

# CHAPTER 12

# Concluding Remarks

Our goal for this book is to offer guidance and, when necessary, a starting point for the ECP to develop a marketing plan for his or her specific practice. Each ECP's needs will vary according to the local marketplace conditions and practice mission. In all cases, the business goals and objectives established for any marketing program are rooted in the practice mission, which comes from the ECP's vision of how the practice should mature. A well-defined mission will guide how the practice is positioned, what patients to target, and how to develop the strategy for product and service features. These are the three main components of developing a practice brand EYEdentity, one of the primary tools used to develop long-term patient relationships. Once these goals and objectives are defined, you can gather information about the local marketplace specific to your strategic requirements. From this marketplace information, you will learn which patient target groups offer the most potential and are the easiest to reach. By analyzing the characteristics of potential target groups and prior patients, you can choose which marketing tactics and components of the marketing mix to use at different points of your marketing program. Once the marketing plan is formulated, the chance of success is greater when proper implementation is accompanied by establishing financial controls and applying benchmark analysis to your practice's performance. The desired characteristics of an ECP's marketing program follow.[1]

An ECP's marketing program should

Be a proactive, ongoing process.
Help anticipate and control change.
Result in improved performance.
Be considered a long-term investment.
Initiate and guide future action.
Identify and focus on specific groups.

An ECP's marketing program should not

Be a one-time event.
Come from dreams.
Be a third-party's opinion.
Be considered the answer to all problems and deficiencies.
Be a reactive process derived from past experience.
Be decided by predetermined personal priorities.

Three fundamental functions must be achieved to ensure the highest probability of practice success: Satisfy the patients by exceeding their expectations, establish long-term patient relationships to realize the highest possible levels of patient loyalty and retention, and staff must reflect the high level of performance your practice brand EYEdentity is to convey.

First, to satisfy patients and exceed their expectations, you must understand what each patient expects and what each patient perceives as a satisfactory level of practice performance. Once this is understood, you can develop desired *standards of performance* for the staff to use as a benchmark for the significant encounter points that influence the patient's perception of the office visit.

Second, to establish *long-term relationships*, seek alliances with suppliers and referral sources that will influence and refer potential patients. Transaction marketing centered around single-patient encounters that emphasize products should be minimized, replaced with relationship marketing aimed at high levels of service quality to retain a loyal patient base. Consider the cost effectiveness of the marketing tactics shown in Figure 12–1. The

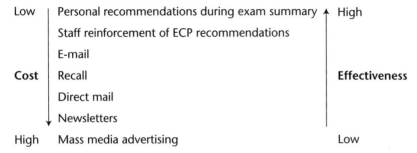

**Figure 12–1   Cost-effectiveness comparison of marketing tactics.**

tactics that cost the least, personal and staff recommendations, probably produce the greatest benefit to both patient and practice revenue.

Finally, train the staff by ensuring all members are aligned with and performing in a manner compatible with your goals. Make sure they possess the skills and knowledge necessary to achieve the high level of practice performance you desire, especially when in direct, unsupervised contact with patients. An improperly or insufficiently trained staff member can undo years of patient relationship building in one encounter. This is an area where small practices may have an advantage over larger corporate and commercial ophthalmic establishments. Practices unable to adequately train ancillary staff members could experience loss of revenue, due to many patients not being served properly and leaving dissatisfied. Staff training and motivation are fundamental elements that could prevent this situation and will be included in the sequel to this book, *Eyecare Business: Management, Motivation, and Finance.*

## Note

1. Modified from Joseph S. *Marketing the Physician Practice.* Chicago: American Medical Association; 2000:8, Exhibit 1-A.

# Marketing Resources

## Market Research

### Sources of Information

- *American Demographics Magazine and Marketing Tools.*
- American Marketing Association: (800-AMA-1150).
- *Burwell's Directory of Information Brokers.*
- Clearinghouse: Find/SVP (212-645-4500).
- *International Directory of Marketing Research Companies and Services.*
- *Trends Journal.*

### Databases

For consumer spending information in your local area go to the Bureau of Labor Statistics website: http://stats.bls.gov.

HomeOwner Data Services
    1270 Turner Road, Suite C
    Lilburn, GA 30047
    (800-326-2368, ext. 122)
    Lists of new home purchases by zip code, addresses, estimated income.

Neighborhood ConnX (888-862-6669) offers small businesses a database that contains demographic information on 90 million households in the United States, updated quarterly.

## Organizations

American Marketing Association
    (800-AMA-1150; http://www.ama.org)
    250 South Wacker Drive, Suite 200
    Chicago, IL 60606-5819
    Provides books, seminars, and publications on database
    marketing. Local chapters also offer their own services.

Direct Marketing Association
    (212-768-7277; http://www.the-dma.org)
    1120 Avenue of the Americas
    New York, NY 10036-6700
    Provides seminars and publications on database marketing;
    sponsors two yearly conferences on marketing.

## Books and Journals

Gaquin D, ed. *2000 County and City Extra*. Bernan Associates
    (800-865-3457); 2000. ISBN 0890592519.
    Includes over 200 statistics for every U.S. county and met-
    ropolitan area.

*Health and Healthcare in the United States: County and Metro Area
    Data*. The Nations Health Company (800-865-3457); 1999.

*Quirk's Marketing Research Review* (612-854-5101).
    A monthly periodical with occasional articles relevant to
    health care; $70 annual subscription.

*The 2000 Research Alert Yearbook*. EPM Communications (888-852-
    9467); 1999. ISBN 1885747241.
    Covers a variety of topics including health care.

Zemke R, Woods J, eds. *Best Practices in Customer Service*. Chicago:
    Amacon (800-262-9699); 1999.

## Benchmark Comparison Data Banks

American Society of Internal Medicine
Internal Medicine Center for Advance Research and
Education
2011 Pennsylvania Ave, NW, Suite 800
Washington, DC 20006-1808
(202-835-2746, ext. 253)
Publishes *Anatomy of Patient Satisfaction: A Primer*, including
survey tools.

Compare2 (800-677-7621; http://rmahg.org) business analysis
software that allows the user to make comparisons to others in the same industry based on the Robert Morris
Annual Statement Studies.

HCFA Database. IntelliMed (phone: 602-230-0333; fax: 602-
280-8909; www.intellimed.com) offers statistical market
research on patient populations. Gaps in different locales
can be determined for potential marketing segments.

Medical Group Management Association:
(877-ASK-MGMA; www.mgma.com).

### Internet Sources

Best practices in customer service:
www.npr.gov/library/papers/benchmark/lstpcus.html.

Best practices/Patient care: www.far.npr.gov/BestP.html.

*Cost and Quality Journal*: www.cost-quality.com.

Joint Commission Accrediting Healthcare Organizations, for
information on performance measurements:
www.jcaho.org/mainmenu.htm.

Links to documents and references: www.qserve.com/hcass.

U.S. Agency for Healthcare Research and Quality:
www.ahrq.gov/data/hcup/hcupnet.htm.

## Books and Articles on Quality and Satisfaction

Berry L. *Discovering the Soul of Service: The Nine Drivers of Sustainable Business Success.* New York: Free Press (800-223-2336); 1999.

Dutka A. *AMA Handbook for Customer Satisfaction.* Lincolnwood, IL: NTC Publishing; 1995. ISBN 0844235865.

Gitomer J. *Customer Satisfaction Is Worthless, Customer Loyalty Is Priceless.* Austin, TX: Bard Press; 1998. ISBN 188516730X.

Johnson M, Gustafsson A. *Improving Customer Satisfaction, Loyalty, and Profit.* San Francisco: Jossey-Bass Publishers (888-378-2537); 2000. ISBN 0787953105.

Kibbe D, et al. A guide to finding and evaluating best practices health care information on the Internet: the truth is out there? *The Joint Commission Journal on Quality Improvement.* December 1997;23(12):678–689.

Sherman S. *Total Customer Satisfaction.* San Francisco: Jossey-Bass Publishers (888-378-2537); 1999. ISBN 0787943924.

Troy L. *Almanac of Business and Industrial Financial Ratios.* Englewood Cliffs, NJ: Prentice-Hall; 1999.

# Information on Marketing and Other Strategy

## Marketing Strategy Books

Kotler P. *Kotler on Marketing.* New York: Free Press; 1999.

Timmins J. *New Venture Creation.* Boston: Irwin Publishers; 1999.

Williamson S, Stevens R, Louden D, Miglone H. *Fundamentals of Strategic Planning for Healthcare Organizations.* Haworth Press (800-342-9678); 1998.

**Website**

Customer relationship management information: www.crm-forum.com.

**Database and Direct Mail Marketing Information**

Gnam R. *Direct Mail Workshop*. Englewood Cliffs, NJ: Prentice-Hall; 1990. ISBN 0137734336.

Hughes AM. *The Complete Database Marketer*. Chicago: Probus Publishing Co.; 1991.
Details how to build a marketing database and use it both to find new customers and to build customer loyalty.

Target Smart! (www.targetsmart.com) software permits you to track purchasing patterns of your best and frequent consumers and direct your marketing efforts to augment these patterns.

To learn about frequency marketing: www.colloquy.com.

**Books on Developing a Brand**

Berry L, Parasuraman A. *Marketing Services: Competing Through Quality*. New York: Free Press; 1995.
Quality and brand development and resource guide.

Levinson JC. *Guerrilla Marketing Handbook*. Boston: Houghton Mifflin; 1995. ISBN 0395700132.

Reis A, Trout J. *Marketing Warfare*. New York: McGraw-Hill; 1997.

Reis A, Trout J. *Positioning: The Battle for Your Mind*. New York: McGraw-Hill; 1993.

**Financial Skills Resources**

American Management Association (800-262-9699 for 1- and 2-day seminars; www.amanet.org). Accounting and Financial

Fundamentals for Nonfinancial Executives. American Management Association.

Dixon RL, Arnett HE. *The McGraw-Hill 36-Hour Accounting Course.* New York: McGraw-Hill (800-262-4729); 1993.

Williamson S, Stevens R, Louden D, Miglone H. *Fundamentals of Strategic Planning for Healthcare Organizations.* Haworth Press (800-342-9678); 1998.
Simple to understand, a good reference book written by business school professors. Doesn't dwell on theory but also doesn't offer alternative approaches.

**Practice Sales Databases**
Bizcomps
    P.O. Box 711777
    San Diego, CA 92171
    (619-457-0366)

Done Deals Data
    717 D Street, NW, Suite 300
    Washington, DC 20004
    (800-809-0666)

IBA Market Database
    P.O. Box 1447
    Boynton Beach, FL 33425
    (561-732-3202)

Pratt's Stats
    4475 SW Scholls Ferry Road, Suite 101
    Portland, OR 97225

**Competitor Intelligence Gathering**
Business ConnX (888-862-6669; www.seriousbusiness.com) software that offers a dozen ways to compare your business to your competitors.

Delorme
>2 Delorme Drive
>P.O. Box 298
>Yarmouth, ME 04096
>(800-452-5931)
>Inexpensive software locates your competitors.

MapInfo Desktop (800-327-8627; www.mapinfo.com) layered
>maps help you to find competitors and potential patients
>within a 20-mile radius.

## Employee Selection Test

Connoly JC, Impara JC. *Twelfth Mental Measurements Yearbook.*
>Lincoln: University of Nebraska Press; 1995.
>Summarizes many of the tests used in screening job appli-
>cants for aptitude and skill levels. Includes a brief evalu-
>ation of their effectiveness.

Equal Employment Opportunity Commission. *Uniform Guide-
>lines on Employment Selection Procedures, 1978.* Washington,
>DC: EEOC; 1978.
>Provides guidelines on how to comply with federal
>employment legislation.

## Sources of Ophthalmic Supplements

This list is strictly for information; it is not meant to be an endorse-
ment of any brands or products.

Body Wise International (714-505-6121; www.bodywise.org),
>Carlsbad, CA, makers of OptimEyes for an aging population.

Interior Design Nutritionals (IDN; 801-345-7420; www.idn.com),
>subsidiary of NuSkin, Provo, UT, makers of LifePak and
>ocular antioxidants.

Rexall Showcase International, subsidiary of Rexall Sundown
>(561-994-2090; www.rexall-showcase.com), Boca Raton, FL,
>makers of Vision Essentials.

Science-Based Health (888-433-4726, www.sbhealth.com),
Carson City, NV, makers of OculaRx, MaculaRx, Optic
Nerve Formula.

## Website Development

### Segmenting Your Market

On-line direct marketers that sell third-party lifestyle data:
Claritas; Acxiom.

Website content developer: pathfinder.com.

Media suppliers: uproar.com; unicast.com; mplayer.com.

ISP (Internet service providers) list: http://www.thelist.com.

A legal primer on Internet contests and sweepstakes, website of
Arent Fox:
www.arentfox.com/features/sweepstakes/home.html.

Sources of entertainment to offer on your site: www.yourco.com.

### Telemedicine

American Telemedicine Association:
(202-628-4700; www.atmeda.org).

Office for Advancement of Telemedicine, DHHS/Health
Resources and Services Administration:
(301-443-3376; http://telehealth.hrsa.gov).

## Patient Satisfaction Survey Resources

American Health Consultants
3525 Piedmont Road, Building Six, Suite 400
Atlanta, GA 30305
(800-688-2421)
Publishers of the monthly journal *Patient Satisfaction and
Outcomes Management* also developers of The Health Care
Satisfaction and Outcomes Tool Kit.

Anatomy of Patient Satisfaction
IMCARE
2011 Pennsylvania Avenue, NW, Suite 800
Washington, DC 20006
(202-466-0291, ext. 243)
Explains basics of conducting a patient satisfaction survey
with a questionnaire.

Health Assessment Lab
750 Washington Street, Suite 345
Boston, MA 02111
(800-572-9394)
Offers provider rating forms and a manual on scoring and
interpretation for $89.

Health Outcomes Institute
2901 Metro Drive, Suite 400
Bloomington, MN 55425
Provides surveys and data collection and analysis services
to health care practices.

**Focus Group Surveys**

Marketing Research Association (860-257-4008; www.mra-net.org).
Provides facilitators to perform patient focus group surveys,
cost typically ranges from $2,000 to $5,000.

Yellow Pages, under Market Research Firms.

Go to www.guidestarco.com and click on customer satisfaction.

**Developing Business Strategy**

*Competition and Business Strategy in Historical Perspective 1950–1997.*
Cambridge, MA: Harvard Business School Publishing
(800-668-6780); 1998.

Mintzberg H, Ahlstrand B, Lampel J. *Strategy Safari: A Guided
Tour Through the Wilds of Strategic Management.* New York:

Free Press; 1998.
Describes ten different views on business strategy.

Sloan Management Review. *In Search of Strategy.* Boston: MIT Press (617-253-7170); 1999.

**Influencing Patient Decisions**
Aubuchon N. *The Anatomy of Persuasion.* New York: Amacom; 1997. ISBN 0814479529.

Charvet SR. *Words that Change Minds.* 2nd ed. Dubuque, IA: Kendall Hunt Publishing; 1997. ISBN 0787234796.

Cialdini RB. *Influence: The Psychology of Persuasion.* New York: Morrow; 1993. ISBN 0688128165.

Hogan K. *The Psychology of Persuasion.* Gretna, LA: Pelican Publishing; 1996. ISBN 1565541464.

## Demographic Data Sources

*Demographics USA 2000 County Edition*
Interactive Market Systems, Wilton, CT
(203-563-3000)
Includes per capita income and consumer expenditures, household and occupational characteristics, and employment data.

*Economic Indicators Handbook,* 5th edition, edited by Arsen Darnay.
Gale Group, Farmington Hills, MI
(800-877-GALE; galeord@galegroup.com)
Comprehensive but complex economic analysis of U.S. cities and towns.

*Markets of the United States for Business Planners,* 2nd edition, edited by Thomas F. Conroy.
Omnigraphics, Detroit, MI
(800-234-1340)

These volumes present personal income data by major economic sector for which earnings are derived for 183 market areas of the United States.

*Profiles of America*
Toucan Valley Publications, Milpitas, CA
Statistical information includes an encyclopedia of U.S. cities and towns; 4 regions of the United States covered in 16 volumes.

*The Sourcebook of Zip Code Demographics 2000,* 15th ed.
CACI Publishing
(800-292-2224) Arlington, VA
(800-394-3690) La Jolla, CA
Includes spending potential index, population composition, and business data.

*Statistical Abstract of the United States*
National Data Book
U.S. Census Bureau, U.S. Department of Commerce

## Lifestyle Data Sources

*Consumer USA 2000*
Euromonitor International, London, England
Includes consumer trends in retail, personal finance, and consumption patterns, as well as housing and household product usage.

*The Lifestyle Market Analyst*
SRDS; 2000, Des Plaines, IL
(800-851-7737)
Ranks top ten lifestyles for each town using home life, good life, investing and money, hobbies and interests, sports, health, high-tech, and outdoor life. Includes consumer profiles, community profiles, and segments.

*Places Rated Almanac,* by David Savageau and Jeffrey Loftus
New York: Simon and Schuster; 1997
Ranks communities according to cost of living, transportation, jobs, education, climate, arts, health care, and recreation.

*The Trends Journal*
The Trends Research Institute
P.O. Box 660
Rhinebeck, NY 12572-0660
Phone: (914-876-6700); Fax: (914-758-5252)
Reports trends within the consumer marketplace

www.census.gov
www.state(then add the 2-digit state code).us
(e.g., California would be www.stateCA.us)
Gets to the official state website with many hyperlinks to
useful information.

# Index